THE COCONUT OIL CURE

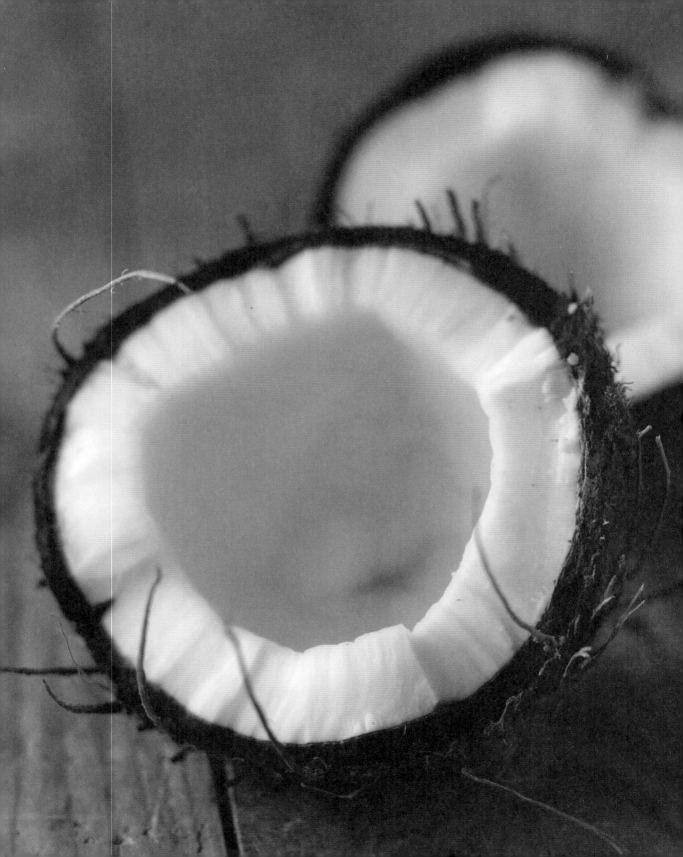

The
COCONUT OIL CURE

Essential Recipes and Remedies
to Heal Your Body Inside and Out

SONOMA
PRESS

TRADEMARKS: Sonoma Press and the Sonoma Press logo are trademarks or registered trademarks of Callisto Media Inc. and/or its affiliates, in the United States and other countries, and may not be used without written permission. All other trademarks are the property of their respective owners. Sonoma Press is not associated with any product or vendor mentioned in this book.

FRONT COVER PHOTOGRAPHY © Stocksy/Sara Remington; Stocksy/Noemi Hauser; Stockfood/Rua Castilho; Stocksy/Aleksandra Jankovic; Stockfood/Tanya Zouev; Stockfood/Gareth Morgans. BACK COVER PHOTOGRAPHY © Shutterstock/images72; Stocksy/Alexandru Sava; Stocksy/Zoran Djekic; Stocksy/Ina Peters. INTERIOR PHOTOGRAPHY © Stocksy/Noemi Hauser, p.2; Stocksy/RG&B Images, p.5 & 12; Stocksy/Aleksandra Jankovic, p.5 & 44; Stockfood/Gräfe & Unzer Verlag / Jörn Rynio, p.5 & 84; Stocksy/Renáta Dobránska, p.6; Stocksy/Zoran Djekic, p.8; Stocksy/Zoran Djekic, p.10; Stockfood/Greg Rannells Photography, p.19; Stockfood/Tanya Zouev, p.34; Stocksy/Katarina Radovic, p.42; Stocksy/Trinette Reed, p.51; Media Bakery/Bernard Radvaner, p.56; Stockfood/Michael Wissing, p.64; Stocksy/Ina Peters, p.82; Stockfood/Michael Wissing, p.91; Stockfood/Laurange, p.98; Stocksy/Sophia van den Hoek, p.104; Stocksy/Sara Remington, p.109; Stockfood/Ian Garlick, p.114; Stocksy/Laura Adani, p.118; Stockfood/Gräfe & Unzer Verlag /Wolfgang Schardt, p.125; Stocksy/Harald Walker, p.129; Stockfood/Valerie Janssen, p.132; Stockfood/People Pictures, p.139; Stockfood/Marla Meridith, p.142; Stocksy/Harald Walker, p.147; Stockfood/Jean Cazals, p.152; Stocksy/Noemi Hauser, p.156; Stockfood/Joseph de Leo, p.163; Stockfood/Alan Richardson, p.168; Stocksy/J. R. Photography, p.172; Stockfood/Gareth Morgans, p.177; Stockfood/Michael Hart, p.181; Stockfood/Rua Castilho, p.184; Stockfood/Rua Castilho, p.192; Stocksy/Sara Remington, p.200; Stocksy/Canan Czemmel, p.207; Stockfood/Valerie Janssen, p.212; Stockfood/Jo Kirchherr, p.219; Stockfood/Valerie Janssen, p.224.

ISBN: Print 978-1-942411-06-2
eBook 978-1-942411-07-9

QUICK-START GUIDE

You might be a coconut oil novice, or you might have a gallon container in your pantry right now for all your cooking and beauty needs. Either way, this book will teach you how to include coconut oil in your daily routine in order to improve your body inside and out. Some parts of the coconut oil journey might interest you more than others, so feel free to jump ahead.

*Learn about the rich history of coconut oil and how the coconut palm is utilized, from roots to leaves. **See page 14**.*

*Get an in-depth look at how an industry war over tropical oil ruined the reputation of coconut oil, and see where that battle stands today. **See page 15**.*

*Read up on the incredible health benefits attributed to coconut oil. **See page 23**.*

*Find recipes for luxurious personal care use and homemade therapeutic applications. **See page 43**.*

*Discover how to cook with coconut oil and coconut products in everything from hot cereals to scrumptious desserts, and every meal in between. **See page 83**.*

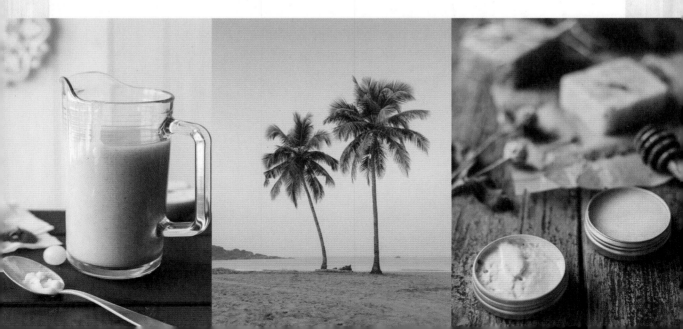

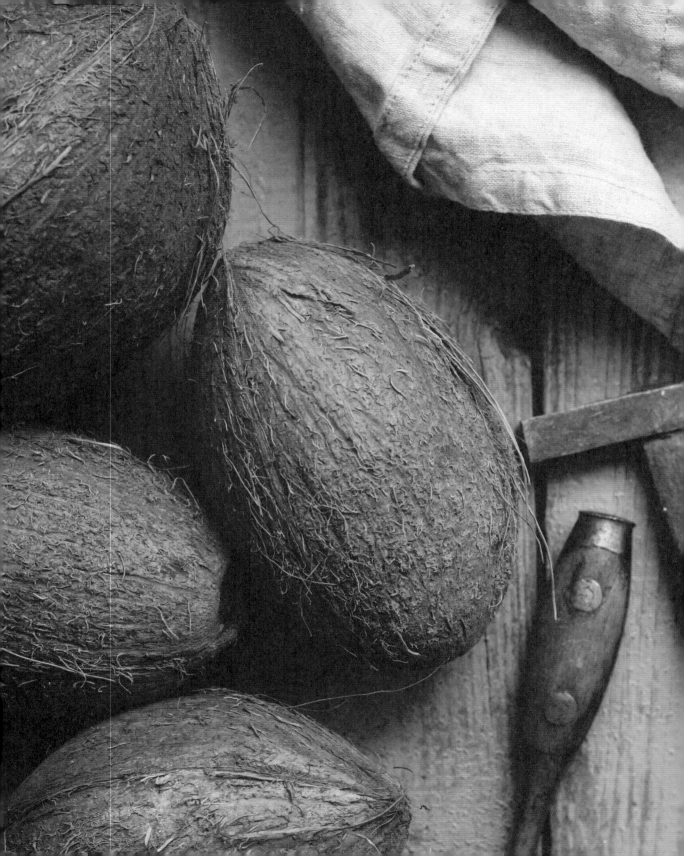

CONTENTS

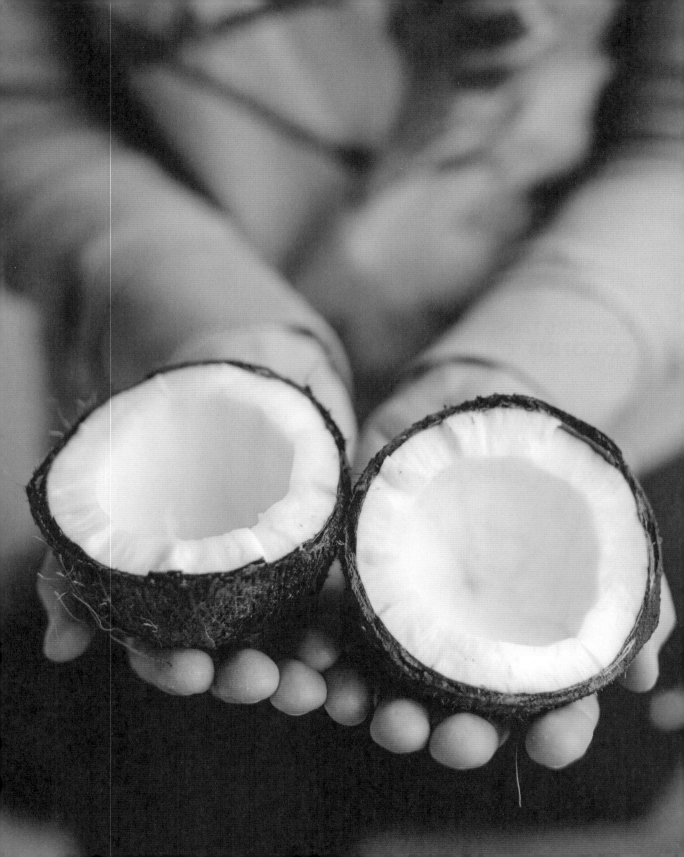

INTRODUCTION

Though it was once regarded as a dietary pariah that led to weight gain and heart disease, these days coconut oil is making a big health food comeback thanks to new research that debunks those old myths, and claims, instead, that coconut oil can benefit your body in a variety of ways, inside and out.

For millennia, cultures across the world have used coconuts and coconut oil as remedies for many different ailments, from skin infections to digestive concerns, thyroid issues, and declining cognitive function. And modern scientific studies have shown that the exotic oil's unique composition of medium-chain fatty acids (MCFAs) can combat bacteria, viruses, and other microbes that can damage your health and cause disease. The fatty acids in coconut oil are easy to digest and boost the metabolism as a quick fuel, and can even help you reach weight-loss goals.

So what can coconut oil do for you? While the Internet is still buzzing with controversy over its ultimate health benefits—offering a mixed bag of skepticism and glowing testimonials—it will do you no harm to experiment with this all-natural (and delicious) product, both in your kitchen and in your beauty routine. Who knows? Whether you try it to whiten your teeth, detoxify your body, smooth your skin, fight infection, or simply add unique flavor to everyday meals, it might just make for a better you.

This book includes everything you need to know about coconut oil and the many ways it can be used to promote good health and overall well-being. Part 1 covers everything from a world history of coconut use to the oil's nutritional components and the essential techniques and equipment needed to create the recipes that follow. Then, in Part 2, you will find 30 easy-to-follow recipes for homemade coconut-oil-based beauty products and therapeutic treatments. And Part 3 will inspire your culinary side with 100 nourishing, coconut-oil-based recipes, including notes that indicate which ones support Paleo, vegan, and gluten-free diet choices.

Are you ready to begin your journey into the world of coconut oil? Let's get started!

Gwyneth Paltrow and Jennifer Anniston swear by it for smooth skin and shiny hair. Emma Stone uses it as a natural makeup remover. Olympic gold medalist Apolo Ohno douses his meals with it to fuel up for big competitions. And celebrity trainer Jillian Michaels cooks with it regularly to boost her immune system and her metabolism at the same time.

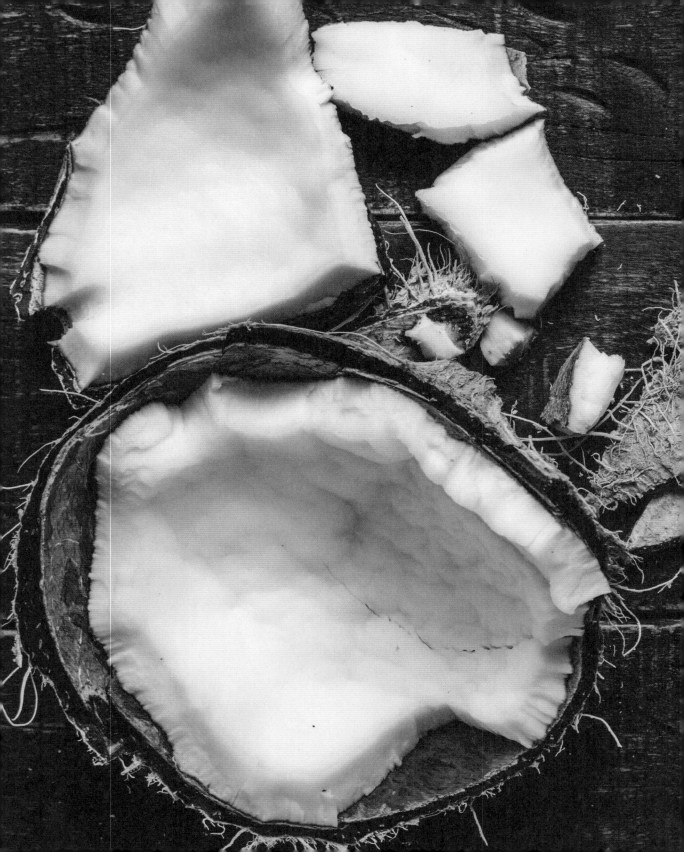

PART I

Understanding Coconut Oil

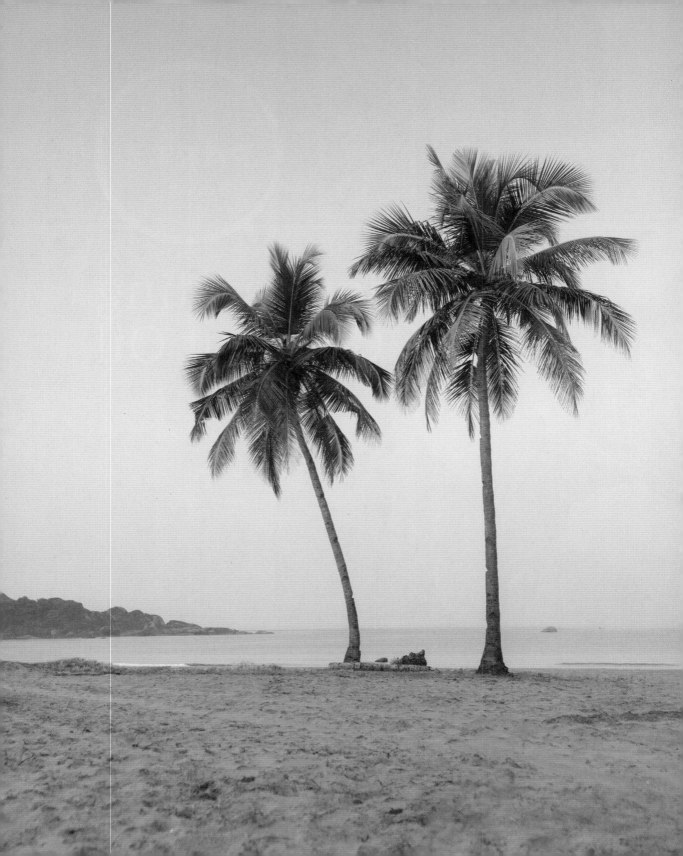

Chapter One

A TROPICAL REMEDY GOES GLOBAL

SCOOP OUT A TABLESPOON of coconut oil and hold it in the palm your hand. As it begins to melt into a clear liquid from your body heat, consider the long, meandering path that led it from the coconut tree to the jar on your counter. Though it may seem unassuming, this rich, snowy-white fat represents a culmination of intricate extraction procedures. And after decades on the "naughty list," it has undergone extensive scientific and nutritional research to rise back into popular favor as a part of a healthy diet. Whether you believe the hype of not, coconut oil is worth a second look.

THE TREE OF LIFE

Often referred to as "the tree of life," for centuries the coconut palm has provided food, shelter, clothing, medicine, and personal hygiene to cultures living in tropical regions across the world. Though it's hard to pinpoint its exact origin, most theories suggest that the coconut first took root in Southeast Asia, from which the buoyant seeds followed ocean currents to other regions in Asia, Africa, Australia, and South America.

The first documented use of coconut oil as a pharmaceutical dates back 4,000 years to an ancient Ayurveda text describing the many health benefits of this tropical elixir. In Ayurveda, a system of traditional Indian medicine, coconut oil is thought to increase strength and nourish the body, and it was used (and is still used today in modern Ayurvedic practice) to soften skin and hair and to protect against skin infections, heart disease, and head lice, among other afflictions. In China, historical documents over 2,000 years old outline 69 different diseases that can be treated and cured by using coconut oil. Anywhere the coconut palm flourished, the local culture utilized coconut oil and other products from the tree for healing and daily life.

Historically, coconut oil has been commonly used for:

- Abscesses
- Asthma
- Baldness
- Bronchitis
- Bruises
- Burns
- Candle making
- Colds
- Constipation
- Cosmetic base
- Cough
- Deodorant
- Dropsy
- Dry and damaged hair
- Dry skin
- Dysentery
- Earache
- Fevers
- Flu
- Fuel
- Gingivitis
- Gonorrhea
- Heart issues
- Heartburn
- Irregular or painful menstruation
- Jaundice
- Kidney stones
- Lice
- Malnutrition
- Nausea
- Oral health
- Perfume
- Rash
- Scabies
- Scars
- Scurvy
- Skin conditions
- Soap
- Sore throat
- Spiritual ceremonies
- Sunburn
- Swelling
- Syphilis
- Tuberculosis
- Tumors
- Typhoid
- Ulcers
- Upset stomach
- Weak bones
- Weakness
- Wounds

"He who plants a coconut tree plants food and drink, vessels and clothing, a habitation for himself, and a heritage for his children."
—SOUTH SEAS PROVERB

It wasn't until the 13th century that coconuts were introduced in Europe. During the Age of Exploration, the hairy, exotic fruits were brought home by adventurers who sailed to South Asia, Africa, and the Americas to forge new trade routes and claim new lands. On their long and treacherous journeys home, explorers and their crew members found that coconuts were much more than simple souvenirs, and they came to depend on these fruits for nutrition and hydration. Over time, the Western world accepted coconut into their various cultures and cuisines, and discovered the healing and medicinal properties that the East had been practicing since ancient times.

THE TROPICAL OIL WAR

Though it has recently re-emerged as a darling of the health food world in the United States, for a brief time coconut oil was cast as a villainous fat—said to cause clogged arteries, spikes in cholesterol, and heart attacks. So how did it fall out of favor, and what brought it back into the public's (and scientists') good graces?

Up until the 1950s, coconut oil was a common ingredient in kitchens and food manufacturing businesses across North America, as well as in beauty products and homeopathic remedies. However, in the 1960s and early '70s, scientific studies revealed that some saturated fats could raise cholesterol levels and therefore increase the risk of heart attacks. Taking this general statement one step further, an American medical researcher, Dr. Ancel Keys, proclaimed that coconut oil was unhealthy because it contained heart-attack-causing saturated fat. He followed this sweeping condemnation of coconut oil with a paper in 1987 that used statistics gathered from seven countries to support his claim; it didn't seem to matter that none of these countries consumed coconut oil. Since over 90 percent of coconut oil's fats are saturated—and further research did not yet exist on the nuances of different saturated fats—this research labeled coconut oil as a health hazard, and soon the public turned against it, opting instead for unsaturated fats such as soybean, olive, and vegetable oils.

Grasping the opportunity to secure its market share in the $3 billion per annum vegetable oil industry in the United States, the American Soybean Association (ASA) swept in with a national smear campaign targeting tropical oils. The ASA distributed a "Fat Fighter Kit" to soy farmers in the United States that instructed them to write protest letters to government and food manufacturers, proclaiming that tropical

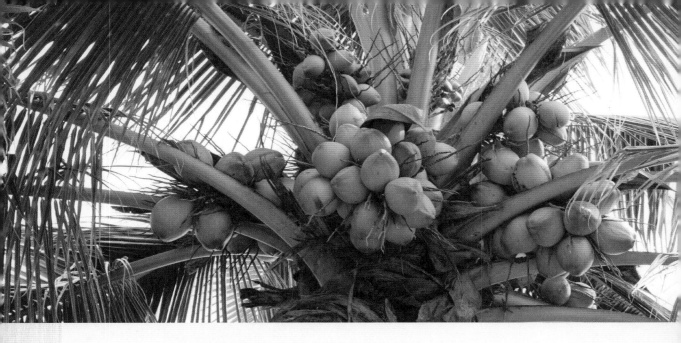

Cracking the Coconut

Coconut trees are found in tropical areas with sandy soil and thrive with plenty of sunshine and rain. Their graceful, ringed trunks soar as high as 80 feet and are topped with crowns of large, feathery leaves. Coconut trees produce a hard-shelled drupe (stone fruit) that is surrounded by a fibrous husk. When it is grown for commercial use, all parts of the coconut tree can be used for many different purposes:

Roots: Used medicinally to treat digestive issues such as dysentery and diarrhea; frayed to use as toothbrush bristles; used in mouthwash and dyes

Trunk: Processed into wood products for construction; ground into pulp to make paper

Leaves: Used by tropical populations as roofs and crude fencing; made into fans, shades, baskets, hats, clothing, and bags; dried and used to make brooms; ground into pulp to make paper

Flowers: Nectar can be boiled down into syrup and used to create alcohol and vinegar

Husk: Used to make rope, rugs, twine, mats, clothing, and as an organic additive to potting soil.

Shell: Used to create utensils, dishes, buttons, and handicrafts; also makes excellent charcoal

Meat / Nut: Eaten raw or dried, ground into flour, shredded, flaked, and desiccated; used as a base for many beauty products

Water: Used for hydration and to replenish electrolytes, enzymes, sugars, vitamins, minerals, and amino acids in the body

Milk: Used to make desserts, soups, sauces, casseroles, and beauty products

Cream: Used in desserts and savory cooking or as a dairy cream substitute

Oil: Used for medicinal, culinary, and industrial applications

oils caused heart attacks. The families of these farmers were encouraged to lobby across the United States, 400,000 strong, extolling the virtues of soybean oil. About this time, several public interest groups such as the Center for Science in Public Interest (CSPI) jumped into the smear campaign by issuing press releases calling coconut oil artery-clogging fat. This group was not yet educated in the structural differences between different saturated fats, so they did not understand that the MCFAs in coconut oil were actually less harmful than the long-chain fatty acids in other vegetable oils. When CSPI released a booklet called *Saturated Fat Attack*, it was called into question by respected researcher Mary G. Eing, Ph.D, who found it full of mistakes. Her protest fell on deaf ears.

These virulent attacks against coconut oil swiftly demoted the oil from revered health food to harmful toxin in the eyes of the American public. Tropical oils were shunned, and foods with unsaturated fats such as salmon, nuts, avocado, and vegetable oils were the only fats that were considered for a healthy diet. Soybean oil topped the list of "healthy" unsaturated oils with no consideration for the fact that these oils are unstable and could get rancid easily. To offset this spoiling issue, manufacturers made soybean oil more stable using a hydrogenation process, which made the oil solid. This process also creates trans fats, which are incredibly bad for cholesterol levels and infinitely worse than the saturated fats they replaced in the North American food chain.

In the midst of this full-blown, completely unsubstantiated health scare, the exporters of tropical oils attempted to fight back, with little success. Coconut oil manufacturers had no political clout and limited financial resources at their disposal, so coconut plantations suffered staggering losses, and countries that depended on coconut products for their economy fell into economic depression. By this point coconut oil had disappeared from grocery store shelves nationwide, but the ASA still wasn't satisfied. In a final push to exile tropical oils from the market, the ASA lobbied the government to bring forth legislation against saturated fat and mandate the use of warning labels on all food products containing these fats. This push for labeling resulted in a series of congressional hearings on the health risks of tropical oils.

Amid all the furor, researchers in the medical and nutritional fields were the lone voices in the crowd announcing that tropical oils did not cause heart attacks. The former US surgeon general, Dr. C. Everett Koop, declared the entire fight against tropical oils foolish, and in

Fun Fact:

The name "coconut" (derived from the Spanish *cocar*, "to grin, make a grimace") is widely attributed to Portuguese explorers who landed in India in the 16th century and were tickled by the fruit's face-like attributes.

1988, Dr. George Blackburn, a Harvard Medical School researcher, testified that groups of people all over the world consumed tropical oils in substantial amounts with no ill effect. Despite this outcry by respected medical researchers, the media and special-interest groups continued to push against tropical oils. Saturated fats were replaced in most restaurants—including fast-food giants Burger King, McDonald's, and Wendy's—with hydrogenated vegetable oils to be "healthier," but in reality this switch doubled the fat content in the food. Soon, almost 80 percent of the vegetable oil used in the United States was soybean oil, and about three-quarters of that was hydrogenated. This saturation of the market by hydrogenated vegetable oils is what actually created the health crisis in the United States, with skyrocketing statistics on obesity and heart disease. Even though research emerged in the 1980s and 1990s that hydrogenated oils raised cholesterol and contributed to many health issues, the myth that discredited coconut oil continued to be considered as fact.

In the early 2000s the research supporting tropical oils as healthful was bolstered by many studies on healthy, vibrant communities all over the world that thrived eating coconut oil. While Americans began to notice the negative effects of the hydrogenated oils they'd been consuming for decades, scientists found that populations consuming tropical oils like coconut oil—instead of hydrogenated oils—had a significantly lower rate of heart disease. This irrefutable evidence made the medical and scientific community back away from their arguments against all saturated fats, and the research continued to pile up supporting tropical oils. For example, a very well respected report published in the *American Journal of Clinical Nutrition*, following more than 350,000 people over 23 years, concluded that there was no connection between the risk of heart disease and consuming saturated fats. The size of the fatty acid molecule became important, and MCFAs in coconut oil were found to decrease the risk of heart disease, while the long-chain fatty acids prevalent in most fats consumed by North Americans were linked to increased cholesterol levels.

The debate over coconut oil's true health benefits and potential risks still continues, but that has not kept this tropical fat from reaching a wide audience in the US health food community. As its popularity grows, fueled by glowing testimonials and health claims from professionals nationwide, coconut oil has become the subject of more and more scientific research, both questioning and touting its benefits.

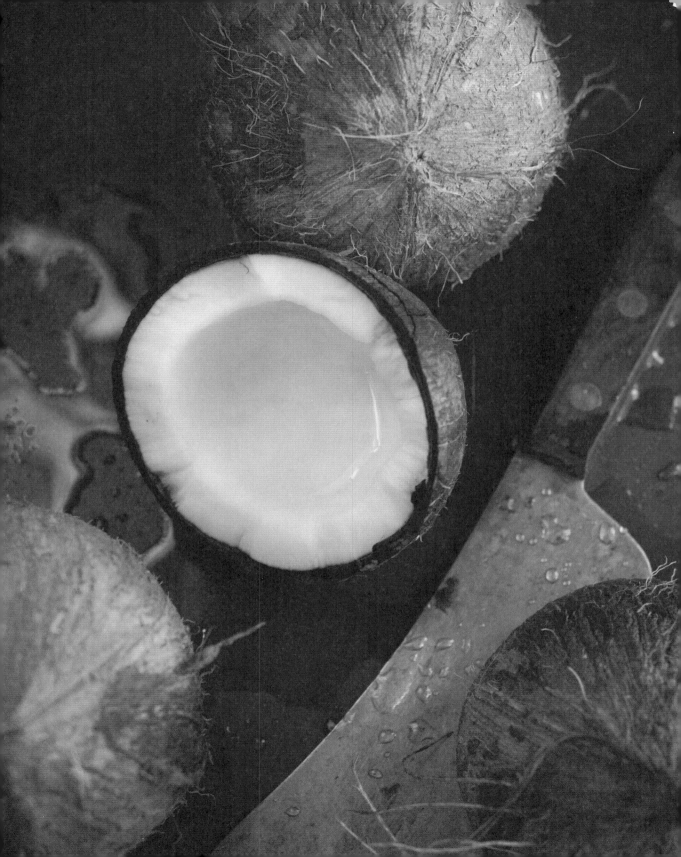

Though scientists have quelled the old claims that coconut oil will clog your arteries and increase your risk of heart disease, they are still determining if the oil can stave off disease or help you lose weight. What scientists will say is that, when taken in moderation, coconut oil will do you no harm. And considering that this natural oil has been used for millennia to remedy all kinds of ailments in cultures all over the world, it's likely that science will catch up to it one of these days.

COCONUT OIL TODAY

Currently, coconut oil can be found in almost every supermarket and health food store across the country, and the Internet brims with success stories and celebrity-backed campaigns touting the oil's many health and beauty benefits. Scientists have also begun to affirm some of the supposed healing properties of coconut oil. For instance, in 2008 the National Library of Medicine released a study indicating that the MCFAs in coconut oil can boost the metabolism and aid in weight loss. This endorsement and various other studies caused a huge surge in coconut oil popularity, increasing commercial sales by nearly 800 percent between 2008 and 2012. And as clean eating, vegan, raw food, and primal (Paleo) lifestyles gained traction in the health and celebrity communities, coconut oil followed on their coattails, soon becoming a darling of the natural foods movement.

Currently, about 80 countries around the world grow more than 150 varieties of coconut, and in many of these places the coconut oil industry is a huge part of the local economy. The countries that produce the most coconut oil or exported copra (dried coconut meat) include Côte d'Ivoire, Fiji, Ghana, India, Indonesia, Malaysia, Mexico, Mozambique, Nigeria, Papua New Guinea, the Philippines, Samoa, the Solomon Islands, Sri Lanka, Tanzania, Thailand, Tonga, Vanuatu, and Vietnam.

It requires a great deal of time and patience to cultivate coconut trees that produce the mature fruit needed for oil extraction. Once the seedlings are planted, they will grow for five years before bearing fruit and another ten years before they reach their full fruit-bearing capacity (about 50 coconuts per year). Then, it takes an entire year for the fruit to mature enough to be harvested for oil.

After the coconuts are harvested, there are several different methods that can be used to extract their oils; the extraction method will determine the quality and purity of the oil, as well as whether it can be classified as virgin (pure) or refined (bleached and deodorized). The most commonly used oil extraction techniques are as follows:

Cold pressed: The coconut meat is dried at low temperatures (103ºF to 180ºF), and then the oil is pressed out. The low heat leaves the nutrients and enzymes intact. Cold-pressed oils are typically unrefined or virgin.

Aqueous processing: Fresh coconut meat is boiled in water until it softens and releases the oil, which then rises to the surface of the water. This extraction technique produces lower-quality oil because antioxidants and nutrients are lost when the coconut meat is boiled. Aqueous processed oils are typically unrefined or virgin.

Centrifuge: Fresh coconut meat is chopped and then transferred to a screw press, which extracts the coconut milk. The coconut milk is then placed in a high-speed centrifuge that separates the oil from the liquid. The virgin coconut oil produced using this extraction method is one of the most expensive, and since no heat is applied during the process, it can be considered a raw product.

Expeller method: Fresh coconut meat is pulverized in a mechanical barrel and pressed into a cake using heat. This cake is then crushed using a rotating rod, and a chemical solvent is added, usually hexane, to separate the oil from the cake. Once the oil is extracted, it is filtered, washed, and bleached. This type of oil is labeled RBD (refined, bleached, deodorized). The finished oil produced with this method will vary in quality depending on the chemicals used and the amount of heat applied to the meat.

Most of the coconut oil used for cooking, therapeutic, and cosmetic application is virgin or unrefined oil because it is considered to be less processed and more healthful. Virgin coconut oil is a very attractive choice for vegans, raw food enthusiasts, and people who embrace a Paleo or Primal lifestyle. Coconut oil is also popular among these groups because it is a saturated fat from a vegetable source that produces stellar results in all culinary applications. To learn more about the different types of coconut oil, see page 36.

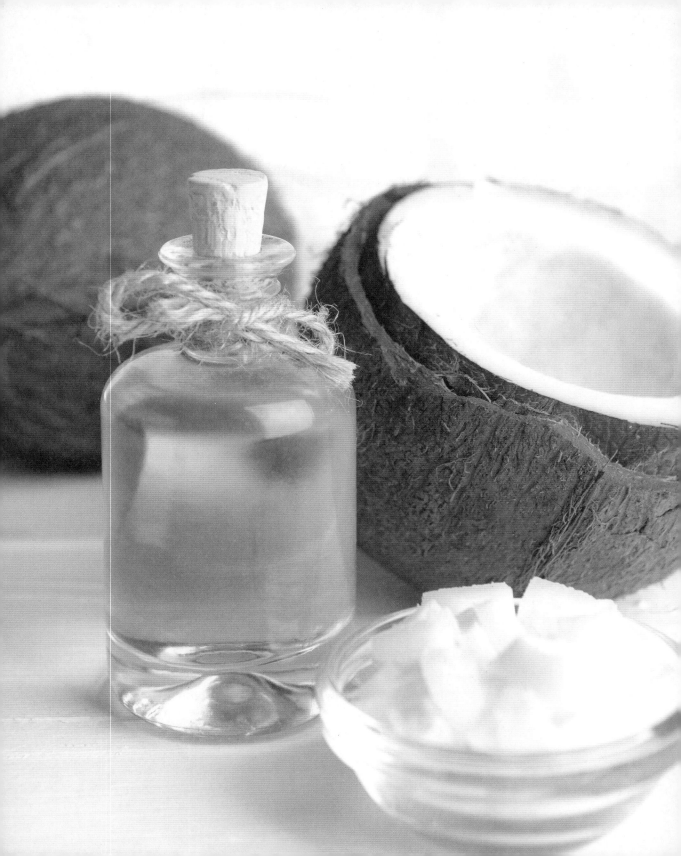

Chapter Two

A MEDICAL "MIRACLE"?

NOW THAT YOU KNOW where coconut oil comes from, how it is extracted, and the history behind the hype, it's time to examine the health claims and testimonials that have elevated this oil to celebrity status in the health and natural foods communities. In this chapter, you'll learn about the nutritional makeup of coconuts, the different health and beauty benefits associated with coconut oil, and the pros and cons of making coconut oil a part of your lifestyle.

COCONUT COMPONENTS

Coconut oil is considered to be a "functional food" because it can provide a bevy of health benefits beyond its nutritional profile. For instance, though it is high in saturated fat—1 tablespoon contains 12 grams—the saturated fat it contains is made up of MCFAs, which are easily processed in the body and can help regulate cholesterol levels and even boost the metabolism.

Once they are introduced in the body, MCFAs are quickly broken down into individual fatty acids and then shuttled to the liver, where they are burned for fuel. This quick conversion to energy helps the body's cells function more efficiently, speeds healing, and gives the immune system a boost. For these reasons, MCFAs are commonly used by hospitals in formulas to treat underweight infants and people with malabsorption issues.

The most prevalent MCFA in coconut oil is lauric acid, an essential component of breast milk that is known to fight bacteria and infection. In the body, lauric acid is converted to monolaurin, a powerful monoglyceride with antiviral, antimicrobial, and antifungal properties. According to a study conducted by the Centers for Disease Control in 1982 and published in the *Journal of Food Safety*, monolaurin can destroy viruses by attacking the lipid-based membranes that surround them. And in further tests, this compound was proven effective against many different viruses and bacteria, including measles, herpes, influenza, hepatitis C, mononucleosis, listeria, pneumonia, anthrax, and various primary and secondary skin infections.

In addition to lauric acid, which is perhaps its most famous nutrient, coconut oil also contains phytosterols, compounds that can help inhibit the absorption of cholesterol and therefore reduce your risk of heart disease. And that's not all. Coconut oil also helps the body absorb vitamins and minerals; is a good source of vitamin E, vitamin K, and iron; and, due to its antibacterial properties, is commonly used as a topical treatment for skin conditions such as psoriasis, dermatitis, and eczema.

Some of the most significant medicinal uses of coconut oil include:

- Analgesic: acts as a pain killer
- Antibacterial: kills the bacteria that cause diseases
- Anticarcinogenic: the antimicrobial properties in coconut oil can help prevent the spread of cancer
- Antifungal: kills fungi and yeast

The Lowdown on Cholesterol

When people talk about "good" or "bad" cholesterol, they are actually referring to the types of lipoproteins that carry cholesterol molecules around in the bloodstream. Cholesterol itself is a waxy substance manufactured by the body to bolster cell walls, aid in digestion, and enable the production of vitamin D and certain hormones. And though it is essential to healthy bodily functions, too much cholesterol in the bloodstream can cause blockages in your arteries, which can then lead to stroke, heart attack, and other serious conditions.

In order to keep your cholesterol levels in check, your body needs to maintain a balance between these two main kinds of lipoproteins:

LDL (low-density lipoprotein): LDL is associated with "bad" cholesterol because it allows cholesterol to build up in the arteries, potentially causing clots and contributing to plaque, which hardens the arteries and makes them less flexible. This cholesterol can also oxidize, which is damaging to the arteries and contributes to dangerously high fat deposits.

HDL (high-density lipoprotein): HDL is associated with "good" cholesterol because it helps to clear excess cholesterol from the arteries and keeps it moving through the bloodstream, reducing the risk of plaque buildup. It ferries "bad" cholesterol back to the liver, where it is broken down and passed out of the body. One-quarter to one-third of the cholesterol in your blood is HDL, and low levels can increase your risk of cardiovascular disease.

There is also another blood lipid that is usually considered when you have your cholesterol tested—triglycerides. If you have high triglycerides, it usually coincides with high total cholesterol levels (high LDL and low HDL) and could indicate diabetes, atherosclerosis (the hardening of arteries) or heart disease. Triglycerides can also be elevated due to a high-carb diet, smoking, obesity, limited exercise, and excessive alcohol consumption.

Ironically, the same saturated fats that were vilified in coconut oil in the past are now heralded as safeguards against cardiovascular disease and other conditions. About half of coconut oil's saturated fats are made up of lauric acid, which can improve your total cholesterol profile, reducing the risk of plaque buildup in your arteries and therefore reducing the risk of heart disease and stroke. Studies published in *Clinical Biochemistry* and the *European e-Journal of Clinical Nutrition and Metabolism* showed that coconut oil can improve blood coagulation and antioxidant status, increase good (HDL) cholesterol levels, and decrease bad (LDL) cholesterol and triglyceride levels.

- Anti-inflammatory: can fight inflammation and block intestinal flora that causes inflammation
- Antimicrobial: the MCFAs in coconut oil are the same as those found in human breast milk. The MCFAs can deactivate harmful microbes while having no effect on beneficial bacteria in the body.
- Antioxidant: protects against free radicals
- Antiparasitic: protects against parasites
- Antiprotozoal: kills a common protozoan infection called giardia
- Antiretroviral
- Antiviral

When shopping for coconut oil, note that the amount of fatty acids in both refined and virgin coconut oil is the same, but the phytonutrient content is less in refined oils. Phytonutrients act as antioxidants in the body, fighting the free radicals that cause inflammation and disease—so, if you want more antioxidant power, stick to virgin coconut oils.

"NATURE'S MARVELOUS ELIXIR"

If you have the Internet or subscribe to any health magazines, you have probably heard incredible claims about the miracles of coconut oil. Despite lingering skepticism from scientists and medical profession-als, a substantial and ever-growing number of devotees maintain that this natural oil is a powerful elixir for all sorts of internal and external ailments. Some of the benefits associated with coconut oil include but are not limited to the following:

Improved absorption of nutrients: Consuming coconut oil can improve the absorption of fat-soluble nutrients and minerals such as vitamins A, B, D, E, and K, as well as CoQ10, lycopene, beta-carotene, amino acids, calcium, and magnesium. A 2012 study in the *Journal of Agriculture and Food Chemistry* showed that combining vegetables with coconut oil before ingesting them can result in your body absorbing up to 20 times more nutrients. For this reason, coconut oil is commonly used in hospital feeding formulas for low-weight infants and has been shown to help increase the survival rate, weight gain, growth, and nutrition levels of premature infants.

Thyroid stimulation: While unsaturated fats can interfere with the thyroid's hormone production, the saturated fats in coconut oil help regulate thyroid function and keep the body at a healthy weight. The positive impact of coconut oil on the liver and metabolism also produces a pro-thyroid effect.

Improved cognitive function: When you ingest coconut oil, a portion of the MCFAs are converted into ketones, a source of energy used by the brain. Ketogenic diets have been used for decades as treatment for epilepsy, Parkinson's disease, Huntington's disease, ALS, brain trauma, and even brain cancer. And for those with Alzheimer's, which impedes the brain's ability to access energy from carbohydrates, ketones are an effective alternative energy source that can help reduce the symptoms of the disease. In fact, in 2009 the Food and Drug Administration (FDA) approved a coconut oil–based dietary supplement for the treatment of Alzheimer's.

Improved digestion: Coconut oil has antimicrobial properties, which can control the bacteria, parasites, and fungi that can affect digestion and cause issues such as bloating, ineffective digestion, and irritable bowel syndrome.

Increased metabolism: Since the MCFAs found in coconut oil are shorter and more water-soluble than those in other oils (like olive and canola), they are instantly converted to fuel in the body, causing a burst of energy that improves metabolic activity.

Better oral health: A technique called oil pulling has been used for centuries to detoxify the body and improve oral health. This technique involves swishing coconut oil around your mouth for at least 20 minutes. The antibacterial properties of coconut oil can inhibit the growth of plaque-causing bacteria (streptococcus) as well as bacteria that causes bad breath and gum disease. A 2008 study published in the *Journal of the Indian Society of Periodontics and Preventive Dentistry* recommends oil pulling as an effective technique for improving and maintaining oral health.

Increased immunity to disease and infections: The MCFAs found in coconut oil are about 50 percent lauric acid, which is converted to monolaurin in the body. When you apply coconut oil externally, it forms a layer that can shield the skin from bacteria, viruses, yeast, and fungi. When taken by the spoonful, coconut oil has been shown to kill viruses and guard against bacteria that causes ulcers, throat infections, sinusitis, urinary tract infections, food poisoning, toxic shock syndrome, pneumonia, and gonorrhea. Coconut oil has also been used to treat parasitic and fungal infections, including giardiasis, ringworm, athlete's foot, candida, thrush, and diaper rash.

Shinier, healthier hair: Coconut oil has been used for centuries in many different cultures as a part of a daily hair routine. Because of its low molecular weight, this oil can penetrate deep into the hair shaft to soften damaged hair and replenish the essential proteins required to promote healthy tresses. Massaging your scalp regularly with coconut oil can also reduce hair loss and encourage new hair growth, as well as eliminate dandruff and prevent lice infestation.

Smoother skin and the reduced appearance of fine lines: Coconut oil is packed with antioxidants, which can protect your skin from free radicals and the negative effects of the sun, as well as vitamin A, which strengthens the connective tissues in skin, therefore reducing the appearance of sagging skin and fine lines. When applied directly to the skin, coconut oil creates a protective layer that can block over 20 percent of the sun's UVA and UVB rays. It also allows MCFAs to penetrate the skin and moisturize from within. Coconut oil can kill the bacteria associated with acne, preventing and reducing the redness of blemishes, and its anti-inflammatory properties can help soothe flare-ups associated with eczema and psoriasis.

Stress relief: In a 2015 study published in the *Journal of Experimental and Therapeutic Medicine*, researchers found that virgin coconut oil was as effective as or more effective than medication for relieving stress among the participants. With a subtle, sweet scent and luscious consistency, it also makes for the perfect massage oil. Try gently rubbing it into your temples and down your neck to relieve mental fatigue and loosen stiff muscles.

Reduced appetite: Feelings of hunger can result from a spike in blood sugar levels as well as a diet that does not meet the protein and fat requirements of the body. Coconut oil can eliminate both of those issues by fueling the body effectively and keeping you feeling full longer. Eating as little as one teaspoon of coconut oil can provide more energy than sugary carbs and stop the sugar cravings that can lead to overeating. Studies in the *American Journal of Clinical Nutrition* and the *International Journal of Obesity and Related*

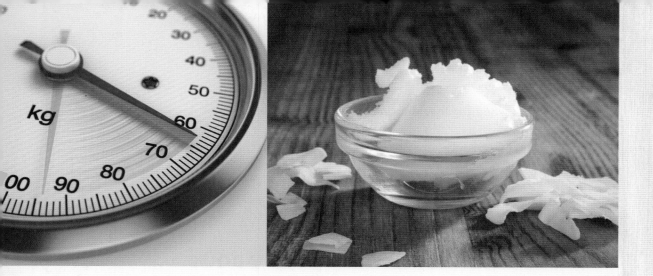

A Fat That Can Make You Skinny?

It may seem counterintuitive, but research has shown that coconut oil and other saturated fats containing MCFAs, when taken in moderation, can help boost metabolism, promote healthy liver function, balance blood sugar levels, and curb hunger—all factors that can result in weight loss. In one study, which was published in the *American Journal of Clinical Nutrition* in 2005, scientists put a test group of 49 overweight men and women on a calorie-restricted diet that included a daily dose of either olive oil or MCFA oil. After 16 weeks, the group that consumed MCFA lost more than twice the amount of weight than those who consumed olive oil. So how does it work?

Since MCFA molecules are short and water soluble, they are sent almost immediately to the liver and converted to fuel, leaving little opportunity for them to be stored as fat. This quick turnaround releases a surge of energy, causing a metabolic increase that in turn prompts the body to burn more calories. It also spurs liver cells to dump their fat content, thereby purifying the liver—the keystone of metabolism—and reducing middle-body fat storage.

Meanwhile, the unique structure of MCFAs in coconut oil can also help you resist the urge to ingest more calories than you really need. The energy these MCFAs supply to the body is equivalent to glucose, but without the blood-sugar spikes and crashes that can lead to binge eating. And coconut oil is just more satisfying than other fats, releasing ketones into the body that help you feel full for longer and reduce your food cravings.

Though science has proven that adding coconut oil to your diet can help you lose weight, this remedy is only effective in combination with other healthy lifestyle choices, such as exercise, stress management, and adequate sleep. To slim down your waistline, first try cutting processed foods from your diet and reducing your sugar intake, then swap out some of your other cooking oils for virgin coconut oil. To take it one step further, some dietitians and healthcare professionals recommend a spoonful of coconut oil in between meals, which can help you curb your appetite and feel satisfied with smaller portions.

Metabolic Diseases show that people who eat MCFAs consume fewer calories per day with no drop in energy or mood.

Improved blood sugar regulation: Coconut oil slows the digestive process so that carbs are broken down less quickly and blood glucose levels remain constant. Therefore, coconut oil can reduce the risk factors associated with type 2 diabetes, such as obesity and insulin resistance. The increase in metabolism created by coconut oil also improves insulin sensitivity and ensures that food is not deposited as fat.

FREQUENTLY ASKED QUESTIONS ABOUT COCONUT OIL

Even if you consume coconut oil daily and include coconut products in every shopping trip, you might have questions about some aspect of this incredible ingredient. Coconut has many uses, and there are many types of coconut oil available. Here are 10 common questions and answers about coconut oil:

How much coconut oil is needed daily for the health benefits?
Coconut oil is not a medication, despite the long list of impressive health benefits associated with consuming it and slathering it on all parts of your body. Therefore, there is no definitive amount recommended by medical professionals as an optimal quantity for health. If you are new to coconut oil, you might want to start with a tablespoon and work your way up to a larger daily dose (up to 3½ tablespoons per day).

Can you experience side effects from eating too much coconut oil?
Coconut oil will not produce side effects, but you can certainly have a reaction to coconut oil if you eat too much all at once or have an allergy. For those who are not used to coconut oil, large doses can result in diarrhea and even some flu-like symptoms. Also, because of its antifungal properties, coconut oil can kill off fungal organisms in the body, leading to a condition called Herxheimer reaction or "die-off." When all these organisms die, they release toxins into the body that can cause fatigue, joint pain, chills, headache, nausea, and swollen glands that can last for several days. If you experience hives, rash, coughing, or swelling of the eyes, throat, or face, it is important that you stop taking coconut oil and seek medical attention.

Can coconut oil go bad?

Coconut oil's unique composition of antioxidants and MCFAs makes it one of the longest-lasting unrefined cooking oils available. However, since it does contain a small amount of unsaturated fats, which break down more quickly than saturated fats, coconut oil will spoil eventually, after about 18 months or two years in the pantry. Avoid using coconut oil that smells off or has changed color.

Can pregnant women use and consume coconut oil?

Pregnant women all over the world have been consuming coconut oil for centuries with no ill effects. Obviously, individuals have different reactions to different foods, so if you are pregnant and coconut oil does not agree with you, then stop consuming it.

Will heating coconut oil impact it negatively?

Coconut oil consists mainly of MCFAs that are not usually altered by the application of heat. Coconut oil will not become hydrogenated when it is cooked even to very high temperatures, because MCFAs are very stable. In fact, heat applied during the production of virgin coconut oil can increase the antioxidant levels in the oil.

Is fresh or dried coconut meat as healthy as coconut oil?

All parts of the coconut have health benefits, but the oil is more concentrated so you don't have to consume as much to reap the health rewards. As little as 1 tablespoon of coconut oil packs in a great deal of antioxidants and lauric acid. In order to get the same amounts of these nutrients, you would have to eat heaps of coconut meat. Coconut meat, however, does contain other nutrients that are essential to the body, such as protein and fiber. This also means that people are more likely to be allergic to coconut meat than coconut oil, because proteins are often the root cause of allergies.

Can you bake with coconut oil?

You can use coconut oil in both solid and liquid form when baking, and it adds a lovely taste and texture to your recipes. If your recipe requires a liquid oil, simply melt the coconut oil and add in the exact same quantity as the original ingredient. Butter can be replaced in a 1:1 ratio with solid coconut oil as well. To substitute solid coconut oil for shortening, use ¾ cup per 1 cup shortening.

Does coconut oil actually taste like coconuts?

This might seem like an odd question, but depending on the kind of coconut oil you buy, the flavor can vary significantly. If you have refined coconut oil in your pantry, then you might discover that it has very little taste or smell. This lack of coconut character can be good if you aren't a fan of the taste. However, if you want a mild coconut scent and flavor, use virgin or unrefined coconut oil for your recipes.

Is coconut oil organic?

Coconuts are rarely sprayed with pesticides because the hard shells don't need added protection from pests. This shell is also cracked off in processing and not consumed, so there is very little chance that the meat, oil, or coconut water could be contaminated in any way. For this reason it is not necessary for a coconut grower to apply for organic certification, which is a costly process. Any organic label you might see on a coconut oil product will refer to the ground and environment in which the coconut trees grew. The ground must be free of fertilizers and pesticides for the coconut products produced from it to be considered organic. The bottom line is that organic coconut oils are not necessarily the best coconut oils on the market, and are likely to cost more.

Is coconut oil safe for children?

Children can benefit from coconut oil as much as adults but should be eased into including this ingredient as a regular part of their diet. Children can be susceptible to diarrhea if too much oil is introduced too quickly. Start your children off with a teaspoon and work up to about 1 tablespoon per day for smaller children and about 2 tablespoons per day for teenagers. Check with your pediatrician if you have any concerns.

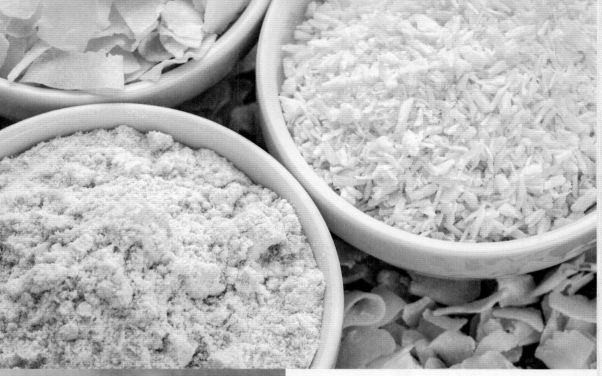

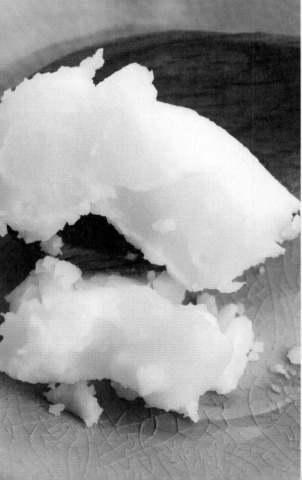

The Popularity of Coconut in Vegan, Paleo, and Gluten-Free Diets

Coconut products are common ingredients in many Paleo, vegan, and gluten-free recipes and sometimes makes up the bulk of calories for people following these lifestyles. Health benefits aside, the attraction of coconut oil, coconut milk, and coconut flour is often due their appeal as substitutes for forbidden ingredients such as dairy products and wheat flour. As a stable source of fat, coconut oil can be substituted one to one with butter for cooking and baking. It is also less expensive than the grass-fed butter some Paleo enthusiasts use in their recipes, and more convenient than rendering tallow from animal products. By cooking with coconut, followers of these diets can still enjoy a wide variety of desserts, breads, ice creams, yogurts, and whipping creams.

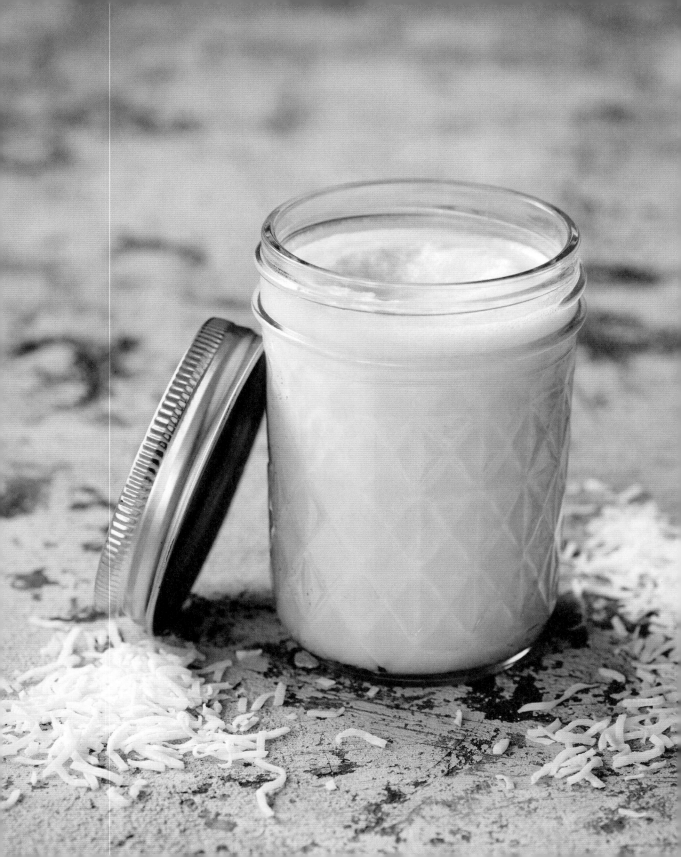

Chapter Three

USING COCONUT OIL

THE DIFFERENT COCONUT OILS on the market vary in extraction method, flavor, price, appearance, and nutritional makeup. So how do you know which one to buy, whether you plan to use it for cooking, weight loss, beauty treatments, or therapeutic applications?

The first step to choosing a specific coconut oil is deciding what type you need. The two basic kinds of coconut oil, unrefined (virgin) and refined, are both rich in MCFAs that can work wonders for your health and beauty needs. However, their contrasting production methods make them better suited for different uses.

The characteristics of unrefined (virgin) and refined coconut oil are as follows:

Unrefined coconut oil

- Also labeled as "virgin" or "extra-virgin"
- Higher in antioxidants than refined oil
- Made by pressing fresh coconut without chemicals, using manual or mechanical methods
- Sometimes produced using heat in the extraction process (Heat gives the coconut oil a stronger coconut flavor. If heat is applied or friction from the extraction process creates heat, the oil is not considered to be raw.)
- Has a delicate coconut scent and flavor
- Is considered to have more health benefits than refined oil
- Best for cooking, beauty, therapeutic, and health applications

Refined coconut oil

- Tasteless, odorless, and with a higher smoke point than unrefined coconut oil
- Contains the same amount of beneficial MCFAs as unrefined oil
- Produced from dried coconut and then refined, bleached, and deodorized (RBD)
- A viable choice if extracted without chemicals using methods such as centrifuge, cold pressing, or expeller pressing
- Less expensive than unrefined coconut oil
- Best for deep frying, soap making, and bath oils

Once you've determined which type of coconut oil you'd like to buy, you might be overwhelmed by the many brands that are now available. To narrow it down, here are a few things you should look for when buying coconut oil:

Container: Though some coconut oils come in plastic containers, clear glass is superior because it will not transfer any taste to the oil, and it has a better seal.

Flavor: You won't be able to determine this until you get the oil home; different brands of unrefined and refined coconut oils may have subtly different flavors. Try tasting a few kinds to determine what coconut oil is your favorite. You might even want to keep a few on hand for different applications: for instance, a flavorless one for general cooking applications, and a more aromatic one for hair and skin treatments.

Price: Unrefined (virgin) coconut oil is more expensive than refined coconut oil. Whether buying refined or unrefined, shop around for the best price, and when you find a brand you like, consider buying it in bulk.

Color: Coconut oil should be pure white when solid, and clear when liquid. Do not purchase or use coconut oil that is discolored.

Organic: Coconuts are not genetically modified or sprayed with pesticides. If a pesticide is used—and this practice is rare—it is added to the roots of the tree.

PURCHASING COCONUT OIL

Now that you have decided to include coconut oil in your life, finding the perfect product for your needs can be bewildering. There are multiple brands of coconut oil lining the shelves of local stores, some of which are represented by distributors rather than individual producers. As a result, identical coconut oil products are being sold under different labels. So how do you choose?

Always start with virgin coconut oil, cold pressed when possible, and in glass jars. If you want to avoid the taste and smell of coconut, then choose a refined coconut oil that has been extracted by centrifuge, cold pressing, or expeller pressing. Do not go to the store without researching specific brands online and finding out the source of the oil, how it is processed, and if the coconuts used were fresh or dried (fresh is better). Expensive isn't always superior, and both small and large companies can produce inferior products. Looking at the brand's website can give you a good impression of how their products are produced and what the company stands for.

The following companies produce or distribute some of the best coconut oil products:

- Alpha DME & Premium Coconut Oil
- Artisana Coconut Oil
- Carrington Farms Coconut Oil
- Fresh Shores Extra Virgin Coconut Oil
- Lucy Bee Coconut oil
- Maison Orphee Coconut Oil
- Niulife Coconut Oil

- Nutiva Coconut Oil
- Tropical Traditions Virgin Coconut Oil

In terms of price, it's worth comparing online retailers like LuckyVitamin.com, Vitacost.com, and SwansonVitamins.com with brick-and-mortar shops like The Vitamin Shoppe or your local health food store. Unless you're able to score free shipping by using online coupons or spending a certain amount of money, the prices of online retailers may not always be cheaper.

STORING COCONUT OIL

Coconut oil is very stable and can last for up to two years in your pantry, and even longer if you keep it in the refrigerator. This oil is solid below 76°F, and if you live in an area where the seasons range from cold to warm, you might find your oil changes from solid to liquid throughout the year. This transition between states will not affect the quality and freshness of your oil, so store your oil where it makes the most sense for your needs.

TOOLS AND EQUIPMENT FOR CONCOCTING CURES AND CREAMS

Making the recipes in the next section requires very little special equipment beyond what you are probably already using in your culinary preparations. However, the storage containers you choose for your homemade coconut oil–based cures and creams will be slightly different from the ones you use for food. Plastic containers can release chemicals into your products, so stick with glass whenever possible. The essential equipment required to create the recipes in the cures and creams section of this book includes:

Stainless steel bowls: Since cures and creams are all made in small batches, you will need a few small or medium-size stainless steel bowls. Stainless steel is a nonreactive material, which will not stain or absorb the odor of essential oils like coconut.

Zester: Fresh citrus zest is a lovely addition to many beauty and therapeutic applications. Clean your zester thoroughly after each use so that you don't introduce any bacteria into your creams, scrubs, and lotions.

How to Open a Coconut

You don't need much preparation or equipment to open a coconut. Just pick a likely candidate and bring it home. If you made a good choice in your coconut, you will hear sloshing when you shake the fruit. The juice inside is sweet, and you will want to save it before whacking the coconut open. If you examine your coconut, you will notice that it looks like it has a face. There are two "eyes" that have a seam that runs between them with a "mouth" below. The "mouth" will be the softest area on the coconut and is the logical spot to create a small hole. Using a screwdriver, knitting needle, or some other thin, sharp object, puncture the coconut through the "mouth" and drain the coconut water into a bowl or glass.

The coconut will have a line that runs around the middle, which you will be able to see. Hold the coconut in the palm of your hand so that the

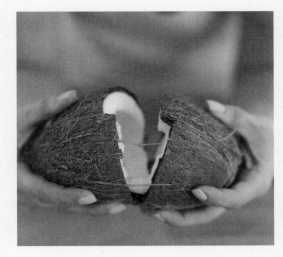

line is in the center and use a mallet or hammer to hit the coconut hard along the line. Hit the coconut about four to eight times while rotating it until the coconut splits open. You can hit the coconut halves until they break into smaller pieces and then use a butter knife or spoon to carve out the coconut flesh.

Hand beater: The easiest and most effective way to make whipped body butters and shaving cream is to beat the ingredients with an electric hand beater. If you use a blender, the coconut oil can melt from the friction, which will ruin the texture of the finished product.

Measuring cups and spoons: Most recipes require you to use exact amounts of different ingredients, so a complete set of wet and dry measuring cups as well as measuring spoons ranging from ⅛ teaspoon to 1 tablespoon is essential.

Whisks: Both small and large whisks are used to beat together the ingredients to create the right consistency for your products.

Silicone ice cube molds: These are great for making massage bars and balms—just spoon the mixture into the mold, then chill until solid. This technique can create gorgeous gifts with professional-looking results.

Containers: An assortment of different-size jars and containers and lip balm holders will be needed to store your lovely products. These containers need lids and should be made of easy-to-clean materials such as glass or plastic.

Spray bottle: You will need a spray bottle to create the hair spray on page 54. The bottle needs to hold at least 2½ cups.

Spatulas and spoons: Many of the recipes in this section are mixed and then transferred to small containers, so spoons are essential tools in your kitchen.

Candy thermometer: In order to get the perfect texture and firmness for your cough drops, you will have to cook your ingredients to a very specific temperature. For best results, use a candy thermometer that clips to the side of the pot.

TOOLS AND EQUIPMENT FOR COOKING WITH COCONUT OIL

You don't need anything out of the ordinary to create most of the culinary recipes in this book, but some dishes require certain appliances to produce perfect results. A kitchen equipped with standard tools is a good place to start, and as you experiment more with coconut oil you may find that you want to add some extra equipment to your arsenal. Here are some tools and appliances that will help you make the coconut oil–based recipes in this book:

High-quality kitchen knives: The first time you use a perfectly balanced, finely honed professional knife in the kitchen is almost a revelation. You cannot imagine the time and energy saved by chopping, slicing, and mincing mounds of vegetables and proteins with a high-quality knife. Hold several kinds in the store to ascertain the most comfortable length, weight, and shape for your hand. Sharpen your knives regularly for best results.

Cutting boards: Safe food preparation requires clean cutting boards designated for meats, vegetables, and seafood. Purchase several sizes of boards to ensure that you have the right board for your needs.

Nested stainless steel bowls: You can never have too many bowls when trying new recipes or preparing family favorites. Stainless steel is a preferred material for kitchen bowls because it is easy to clean and does not stain or rust.

Nonstick cookware: A selection of pots and pans of different sizes and depths can make your culinary life easier. Look for nonstick cookware coated with Thermolon or Sandflow, as these materials are considered safer than others.

Peeler and zester: These tools are convenient for preparing root vegetables and zesting citrus fruits. In order to keep these tools effective, make sure you clean them thoroughly after each use.

Measuring cups and spoons: The success of recipes is dependent on accurate measurements in most cases, so invest in a complete set of wet and dry measuring cups as well as measuring spoons ranging from ⅛ teaspoon to 1 tablespoon.

Whisks: Both small and large whisks are used to beat together the ingredients to create the right consistency for your recipes.

Immersion blender: This is not an essential tool, but it can be used in place of a blender or food processor for some recipes such as soups, smoothies, and sauces. This tool is less expensive than larger appliances, easy to clean, and takes up very little room in your kitchen.

Good-quality blender: You can never go wrong with a powerful blender for your smoothies, ground nuts, and soups. You don't need to break the bank on a blender, but at least find one that can crush ice cubes easily.

Food processor: This appliance is essential for making nut butters, puréeing in large batches, and preparing heaps of sliced or chopped vegetables. Look for a processor with a 10- to 12-cup capacity.

Ice cream maker: You might only make ice cream periodically, but when cravings strike, there is no better way to make it at home.

Waffle maker: Most waffle makers are extremely simple to operate and can also be used to make tasty grilled cheese sandwiches when you aren't making breakfast.

Grill: Grilled proteins, seafood, and vegetables are fabulous, and this cooking technique cuts time and effort in the kitchen. If you do not have the space for a larger propane grill, pick up a small briquette one that works on a balcony or fits in a small outdoor space.

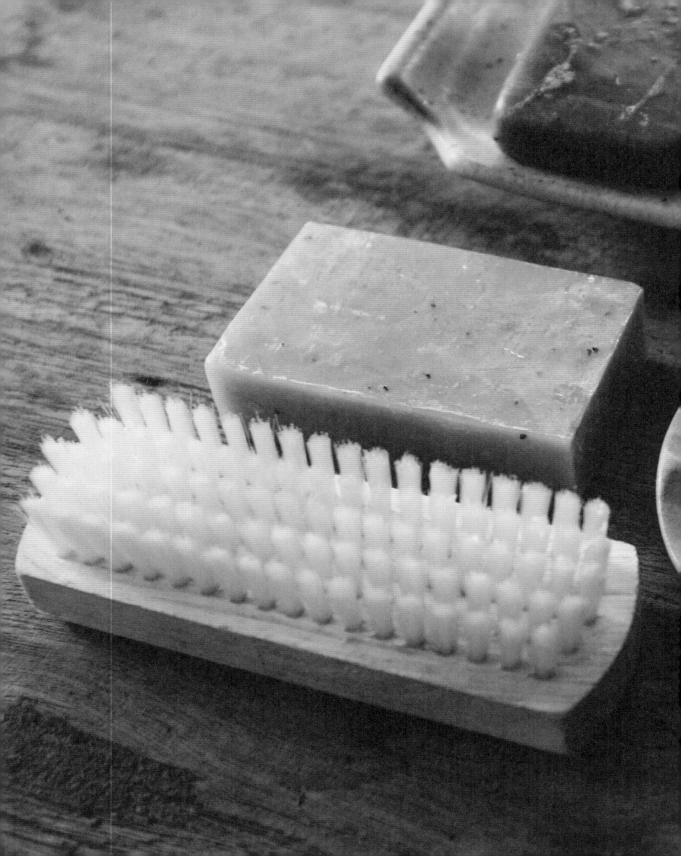

PART II

Cures & Creams

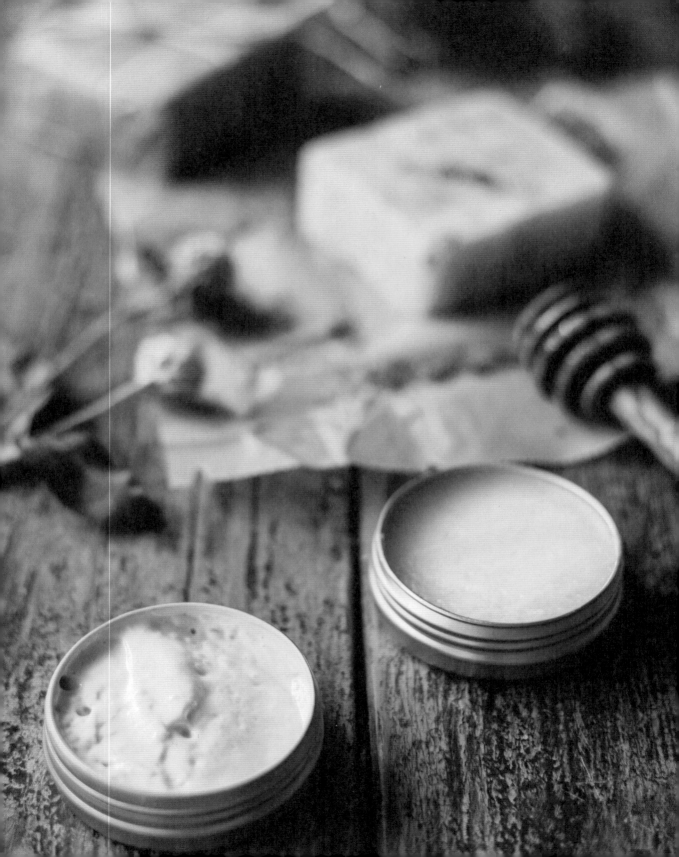

Chapter Four

NATURAL COSMETICS

SWEET VANILLA MASSAGE BARS

MAKES 10 BARS • PREP TIME: 15 MINUTES PLUS CHILLING TIME • COOK TIME: 2 MINUTES

If you are looking for a gift for someone who enjoys a little luxury, these creamy molded massage bars are the perfect choice. Five nutrient-packed oils are featured here to ensure dewy velvet skin without a greasy sensation. Cocoa butter is incredibly high in fatty acids, so it penetrates deeper than the skin surface to hydrate from within. The almond oil can help restore normal PH to your skin while calming inflamed areas. If you suffer from stretch marks or want to smooth chronic chapped elbows or knees, double this recipe so you'll always have a solution on hand.

½ cup coconut oil

½ cup shea butter

2 tablespoons grated cocoa butter

2 teaspoons sweet almond oil

½ teaspoon vitamin E oil

12 drops vanilla essential oil

1. Set a small saucepan of water over medium-low heat and place a small stainless steel bowl on the top of the saucepan so that the bottom is just above the water. Bring the water to a gentle simmer and reduce the heat to low.

2. Add the coconut oil, shea butter, and cocoa butter to the bowl and stir until it is melted, about 2 minutes.

3. Remove the bowl from the top of the saucepan and stir in the almond oil, vitamin E oil, and vanilla essential oil until the mixture is smooth.

4. Spoon the mixture into pretty silicone bar-shaped molds (or ice pop molds) and let it cool until hardened, about 1 hour.

5. Remove the bars from the molds and store them in a sealed jar in the refrigerator until you want to use them, for up to 3 months.

TIP When you want a fragrant, nourishing massage, remove a lotion bar from the refrigerator and hold it in your closed hand until it softens. The oils in the bar will melt at body temperature, so it will not take long to get the right texture for a massage. You can also run the chilled lotion bar over your skin, or someone else's, and let the friction and heat from the body melt the bar as you proceed.

SOOTHING MILK BATH

MAKES 2 CUPS • PREP TIME: 5 MINUTES • COOK TIME: 0 MINUTES

For centuries, milk baths have been used as a treatment for chapped skin and other conditions. In this version, coconut milk is used instead of cow's milk, to great effect. Rich in restorative vitamin E and skin-penetrating fatty acids, coconut milk protects the skin and provides deep nourishment. The eucalyptus essential oil can help improve your circulation, giving you a healthy glow, and the lavender is a natural antibacterial and anti-inflammatory that helps reduce the appearance of scars and stretch marks.

1 (15-ounce) can coconut milk

6 drops eucalyptus essential oil

6 drops lavender essential oil

Dried lavender (optional)

1. Pour the coconut milk into a jar or bottle.

2. Add the eucalyptus and lavender essential oils and dried flowers if using.

3. Put the lid on your jar and shake until the contents are well mixed.

4. Pour 1 cup of the milk into a running bath and enjoy.

5. Store the remaining milk bath in the refrigerator for up to 2 weeks.

TIP Although it is tempting to run a super-hot steamy bath when you feel like pampering yourself, if your water is too hot it can be extremely drying for your skin. Try having the water temperature at a less scalding level and let the lavender scent, instead of the heat, relax you.

COCONUT-VANILLA SALT SCRUB

MAKES 1½ CUPS • PREP TIME: 10 MINUTES • COOK TIME: 0 MINUTES

Scrubs are an effective method of removing dead skin cells from any part of your body to reveal fresh, glowing skin. If you are applying this sweet-smelling scrub to your face, make sure you use just your fingertips in a gentle circular pattern rather than an up and down scrubbing motion with your palms. You want to buff your skin, not scrape it raw. Epsom salt is not actually salt but a healthful natural compound of magnesium and sulfate that is absorbed through the skin to help detoxify and decrease inflammation.

1 cup coconut oil

½ cup Epsom salt

6 drops vanilla essential oil

1. Mix the coconut oil and Epsom salt together in a medium bowl until well combined.

2. Add the vanilla essential oil and stir until the mixture is evenly blended.

3. Store the salt scrub in a sealed glass container at room temperature for up to 1 month.

TIP   Scrubs are best applied in the shower to avoid a mess if you want to use them all over your body. Take care if you are exfoliating your feet, especially the bottoms, because the coconut oil can be slippery on the surface of the bathtub or shower stall.

ORANGE CREAMSICLE WHIPPED BODY BUTTER

MAKES 2½ CUPS • PREP TIME: 15 MINUTES PLUS 20 MINUTES COOLING • COOK TIME: 2 MINUTES

You might have a difficult time not using a spoon to eat this luscious orange-scented body butter—but please refrain, because it does not taste as good as it smells. The orange oil used in this recipe is also known as sweet orange oil, so make sure you do not pick up the bitter orange product instead. Sweet orange oil is extracted by cold pressing orange peels rather than using steam. This essential oil is a wonderful stress reliever and can brighten up dull skin.

1 cup coconut oil

¾ cup cocoa butter

40 drops orange essential oil

10 drops vanilla essential oil

1. Set a small saucepan over low heat and add the coconut oil and cocoa butter.

2. Stir until melted and well combined, about 2 minutes.

3. Transfer the coconut oil mixture to a medium stainless steel bowl and stir in the orange and vanilla essential oils until well blended, about 30 seconds.

4. Put the bowl in the refrigerator until the mixture is starting to solidify but is not completely solid, about 15 to 20 minutes.

5. Use an electric hand beater on medium speed to whip the mixture until it is very light and fluffy, about 10 minutes, scraping down the sides of the bowl at least once.

6. Spoon the body butter into a container such as a glass jar with a lid.

7. Store at room temperature for up to 2 months.

TIP Some people are sensitive to citrus oils, so try this body butter on a small area first and wait a few hours to see if you have any reaction. Citrus oils can be phototoxic, meaning that they can produce a reaction like sunburn when exposed to light. The amount of sweet orange oil used in this recipe is quite small, but you still should avoid very strong direct sunlight right after applying the body butter.

HONEY-COCONUT SUGAR SCRUB

MAKES 1½ CUPS • PREP TIME: 10 MINUTES • COOK TIME: 0 MINUTES

The sharp lemon fragrance of this scrub will wake you up while you gently apply it to your face or décolletage. Lemon essential oil is very effective at eliminating dull skin and equalizing oily skin. You can use either white or brown sugar for this scrub with similar, silky-fresh results. Raw honey adds a pleasing sweet scent to the scrub while unclogging pores, and moisturizing for a pretty glow. Honey is also a powerful antibacterial agent, which can cut down the frequency of breakouts and reduce the inflammation of existing blemishes.

---

1 cup raw sugar

½ cup coconut oil, melted

2 tablespoons raw honey

1 tablespoon olive oil

10 drops lemon essential oil

1. In a medium bowl, mix together the sugar, coconut oil, honey, and olive oil until well blended. You should make sure that there are no large sugar clumps in the mixture.

2. Add the lemon essential oil and mix until evenly blended.

3. Spoon the scrub into a glass container with a lid, like a glass jar.

4. Store at room temperature for up to 6 months.

TIP Whenever possible, try to purchase steam-distilled lemon essential oil; unlike cold-pressed lemon oil, it is not phototoxic. Read the label on the oil to learn the extraction process or look up the brand online for the information you need.

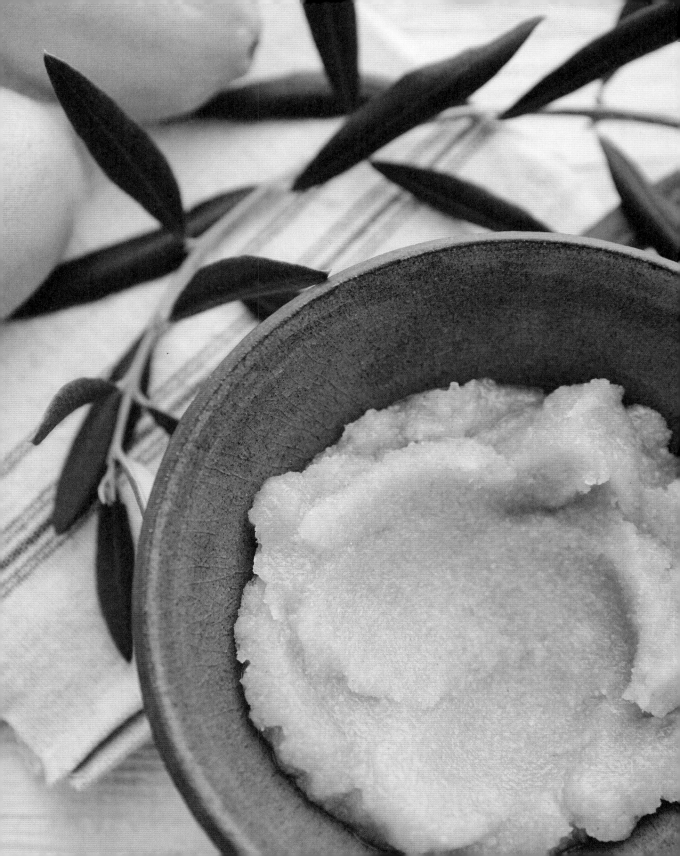

COCONUT FACE CLEANSER

MAKES ¾ CUP • PREP TIME: 5 MINUTES • COOK TIME: 0 MINUTES

You might find it strange to cleanse your face with oil rather than a tingly toner or sudsy soap, but this oil-based cleanser will make your skin feel cleaner and look more radiant. It is a proven fact that like dissolves like, and in this case the dirty oil sitting on your skin is dissolved and removed by the oil in the cleanser. This way, you will wipe away the pore-clogging layer without stripping your skin of its own natural moisture. The neem oil in this cleanser will not only clean your skin; it will also improve your skin's elasticity and protect against environmental damage.

½ cup coconut oil, melted

Juice of ½ lemon

1 teaspoon honey

10 drops neem essential oil

5 drops tea tree essential oil

1. In a small bowl, whisk together the coconut oil, lemon juice, honey, and neem and tea tree essential oils.

2. Transfer the cleanser to a small glass container with a lid.

3. Store at room temperature for up to 2 weeks.

TIP   Pour about 1 tablespoon of cleanser in your palm and gently rub your hands together. Apply the oil generously to your face, avoiding your eyes, and massage into the skin for several minutes. Let the cleanser sit on your face for 5 minutes and then use a clean cloth dunked in very warm water to gently wipe the oil cleanser away. You might have to wring out the cloth once depending on how much cleanser you applied.

COCONUT MILK–YLANG YLANG SHAMPOO

MAKES 1¼ CUPS • PREP TIME: 5 MINUTES • COOK TIME: 0 MINUTES

Solid coconut oil might not look like it could make an effective shampoo, but it lathers up beautifully when used in this fragrant shampoo recipe. Coconut oil and coconut milk nourish hair and promote hair growth while detangling and strengthening. What could be healthier for your crowning glory? The addition of ylang ylang essential oil, which is considered to be an aphrodisiac, adds a lingering, seductive floral scent that is perfect if you are planning a romantic evening. Ylang ylang also promotes an elevated mood and relieves anxiety, so this shampoo is wonderful for everyday use.

¾ cup liquid castile soap

½ cup canned coconut milk

1 tablespoon coconut oil

15 drops ylang ylang essential oil

1. In a medium bowl, whisk together the castile soap, coconut milk, and coconut oil until blended, about 1 minute.

2. Whisk in the ylang ylang essential oil and pour the shampoo into a jar or bottle with a lid.

3. Store the shampoo for up to 1 month, and shake before using.

TIP   If your bathroom gets very cold, you might want to store this shampoo in a warmer area of the house so the coconut oil doesn't solidify between uses. If your shampoo does get too thick, put the bottle or jar in a bowl of warm water until the oil melts again.

COCONUT OIL BEACH HAIR SPRAY

MAKES 2½ CUPS • PREP TIME: 5 MINUTES • COOK TIME: 0 MINUTES

Wouldn't it be lovely to get that tousled beachy look without sand caked to your skin and a painful sunburn? This simple citrus spray will add volume and texture to your hair with just a few spritzes. The coconut oil will ensure that the salt does not dry out your hair, and the hair gel adds exactly the right hold all day. You can omit the gel if you want a completely natural product, but you might have to reapply your spray throughout the day.

2 tablespoons coconut oil, melted

4 teaspoons sea salt

2 teaspoons favorite hair gel

10 drops lemon essential oil

2 cups hot water

Spray bottle

1. In a small bowl, stir together the coconut oil, salt, hair gel, and lemon essential oil until well blended.

2. Whisk in the hot water and pour the mixture into a spray bottle.

3. Shake and spray generously onto damp hair.

4. Store the spray for up to 2 months at room temperature.

TIP You can use beach hair spray on either dry or damp hair with spectacular effects. If you prefer a dry-hair application, make sure this is the last step in your styling process and make sure you do not apply it to your hair's roots. If you apply the spray to damp hair, spritz the ends and mid-length, staying away from the roots, and let your hair dry naturally.

FRAGRANT SHAVING CREAM

MAKES 1½ CUPS • PREP TIME: 10 MINUTES • COOK TIME: 1 MINUTE

Who would have thought you could create frothy moisturizing shaving cream yourself with no damaging aerosol cans or skin-irritating ingredients? In this cream, the frankincense essential oil creates a woodsy, earthy scent that is not overpowering or pungent. If you want a stronger aroma, simply increase the number of drops you use for the cream. The shea butter in this cream will help your razor glide smoothly, reducing the incidence of unsightly, painful razor bumps. Shea butter will also soothe itchy, irritated skin after shaving if you have sensitive skin or used a dull razor.

½ cup coconut oil

¼ cup shea butter

½ cup liquid castile soap

1 tablespoon baking soda

4 drops frankincense essential oil

2 drops lavender essential oil

1. Set a small saucepan of water over medium heat and place a small bowl on the top of the saucepan so that the bottom is just above the water. Bring the water to a gentle simmer and reduce the heat to low.

2. Add the coconut oil and shea butter to the bowl and stir until melted and well combined, about 1 minute.

3. Remove the bowl from the top of the saucepan and add the castile soap, baking soda, and frankincense and lavender essential oils. Stir to combine.

4. Use an electric hand beater on medium speed to whip the mixture to a fluffy texture, about 3 minutes.

5. Transfer the shaving cream to a glass container with a lid.

6. Store in the refrigerator for up to 2 weeks. The cream will harden but can still be used as is or if you whip it again. The shaving cream can also be left out for 3 days at room temperature or used right away.

TIP This cream is best used right away, when it is at room temperature. So if you only have to shave a small area, cut the recipe in half and whip up the cream when you need it. This recipe makes enough for shaving both legs and the bikini area.

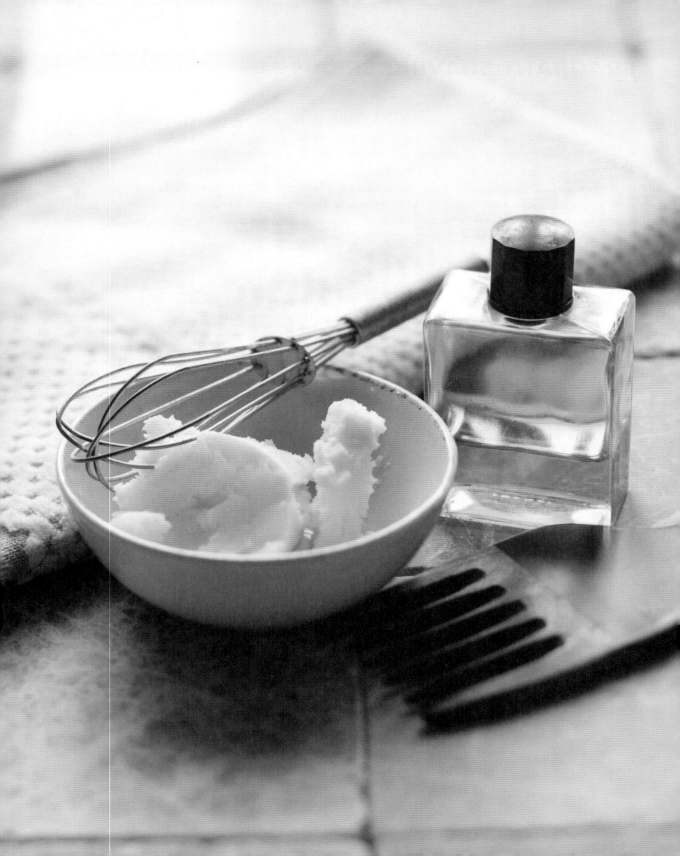

HOT COCONUT OIL HAIR TREATMENT

MAKES ¾ CUP • PREP TIME: 10 MINUTES • COOK TIME: 0 MINUTES

Why spend lots of money on expensive spa oil treatments for your hair when you can whip up this sweet, fruity oil in the comfort of your own home? Roman chamomile can soothe your mood while helping infuse your locks with moisture and promoting hair growth. Do not exclude the vitamin E; it helps prevent split ends and makes your hair stronger and more lustrous. The easiest way to get vitamin E is to buy gel caps and break them open when you need the oil for your recipes.

½ cup melted coconut oil

¼ teaspoon vitamin E oil

10 drops lavender essential oil

10 drops Roman chamomile essential oil

1. In a small bowl, whisk together the coconut oil and vitamin E oil.

2. Add the lavender and Roman chamomile essential oils and whisk to blend, about 30 seconds.

3. Use the oil right away on dry hair starting at the ends.

4. Apply the oil generously on the lower lengths and lightly near the roots. Use a wide-tooth comb to distribute the oil evenly.

5. Clip your hair back and let the treatment sit for at least 1 hour or up to 12 hours. If you want to leave it on longer than 1 hour, wrap your head in a towel or put on a cap.

6. Use a mild shampoo to wash the treatment out.

7. Store the hair treatment for up to 1 week in a sealed jar at room temperature.

TIP Do not apply much of the oil treatment to your hair's roots. Most hair damage occurs at the ends, caused by hair dryers and hot flat irons. It can also be difficult to remove the oil from your scalp without shampooing several times, which will dry out your hair again.

LAVENDER CALMING LOTION

MAKES 1½ CUPS • PREP TIME: 5 MINUTES PLUS 30 MINUTES COOLING • COOK TIME: 2 MINUTES

You will delight in the heavenly fragrance of this lotion and enjoy the lush moisturizing feeling on your skin. Lavender is one of the most popular essential oils for very good reason—the light floral fragrance has an herbal undertone that is well respected for its calming, stress-relieving properties. The beeswax in this lotion will ensure that it does not break down and lose its texture while helping your skin retain its natural moisture. An added benefit of beeswax is that it will not clog your pores, making this a great lotion for those with oily skin.

---

1 cup coconut oil

¼ cup beeswax

12 drops lavender essential oil

1. Set a small saucepan of water over medium-low heat and place a small bowl on the top of the saucepan so that the bottom is just above the water. Bring the water to a gentle simmer and reduce the heat to low.

2. Add the coconut oil and beeswax to the bowl and stir until melted and well combined, about 2 minutes.

3. Remove the bowl from the saucepan and add the lavender essential oil to the melted coconut oil mixture. Stir to blend.

4. Let the mixture cool completely, for about 30 minutes.

5. Use an electric hand beater on medium speed to whip the cooled mixture to a creamy texture, about 1 minute.

6. Transfer the lotion to a glass container with a lid.

7. Store at room temperature for up to 2 months.

TIP This lotion can be used all over your body. Apply it to your skin just before bed to help you drift away into soothing dreams. If you have a bee allergy, it is better to substitute cocoa butter in the same quantity for the beeswax to avoid any interactions.

BRONZING CINNAMON BODY BUTTER

MAKES 2½ CUPS • PREP TIME: 15 MINUTES PLUS CHILLING TIME • COOK TIME: 2 MINUTES

For decades, tanned skin was seen as the epitome of a healthy appearance, but we know now that tanning is incredibly bad for your skin. When your skin is exposed to UV light, it protects itself by producing melanin, and this dark color means that the DNA in your skin has been damaged. So why not achieve that sun-kissed glow using a natural product instead? Cocoa powder and cinnamon are the tinting agents in this luxurious, spicy body butter, and the cinnamon not only tints the outside but also brings the blood to the surface of the skin, creating an extra glow.

---

1 cup coconut oil

½ cup shea butter

½ cup sweet almond oil

2 tablespoons cocoa powder

½ teaspoon vitamin E oil

10 drops cinnamon essential oil

1. Set a small saucepan over low heat and add the coconut oil and shea butter.

2. Stir until melted and well combined, about 2 minutes.

3. Transfer the coconut oil mixture to a medium stainless steel bowl and whisk in the almond oil, cocoa powder, vitamin E oil, and cinnamon essential oil until well blended and very smooth, about 2 minutes.

4. Put the bowl in the refrigerator until the mixture is just solid enough that you can leave an indent in the top with the tip of your finger, about 15 to 20 minutes.

5. Use an electric hand beater to whip the mixture until it is very light and fluffy, about 10 minutes, scraping down the sides of the bowl at least once.

6. Spoon the body butter into a container such as a glass jar with a lid.

7. Store at room temperature for up to 2 months.

TIP This body butter will not permanently stain your skin like chemical self-tanners, but if you let it dry completely, it should not stain your clothes or streak. You have complete control over how dark you want to make this butter, as well. If you are very fair, cut the cocoa and cinnamon amounts in half to create a subtler shade.

MINTY DEODORANT

MAKES 1 CUP • PREP TIME: 5 MINUTES • COOK TIME: 1 MINUTE

Store-bought deodorants, in particular antiperspirants, have had some bad press in recent years because most products contain aluminum and other possibly dangerous chemicals. Aluminum is linked to Alzheimer's disease, kidney disease, and seizures. Making your own deodorant that does not stop the healthy process of toxin-releasing perspiration seems like a healthy solution to underarm odor issues. The arrowroot starch in this recipe is pleasingly silky and effective for absorbing odor. This deodorant uses peppermint, which is stimulating to the senses and produces a lovely cooling sensation.

½ cup coconut oil

3 tablespoons baking soda

3 tablespoons arrowroot starch

1 teaspoon vitamin E oil

15 drops peppermint essential oil

1. Set a small saucepan of water over medium heat and place a small bowl on the top of the saucepan so that the bottom is just above the water. Bring the water to a gentle simmer and reduce the heat to low.

2. Add the coconut oil to the bowl and stir until it is softened, about 1 minute.

3. Remove the bowl from the top of the saucepan and stir in the baking soda, arrowroot, vitamin E oil, and peppermint essential oil until the mixture is smooth.

4. Spoon the deodorant into a small glass container with a lid.

5. Store up to 1 month.

TIP   Use your fingertips to scoop out about ½ teaspoon of deodorant and smooth the paste over the entire underarm area. Repeat for the other underarm. Be careful using this deodorant if you plan to wear a black shirt; it can cause visible white marks on the fabric if you dress before the paste dries on the skin.

PEPPERMINT-COCONUT TOOTHPASTE

MAKES ¾ CUP • PREP TIME: 5 MINUTES • COOK TIME: 0 MINUTES

If you are familiar with the centuries-old oral health ritual of oil pulling, then the idea of making toothpaste out of coconut oil, or any oil, will seem logical. Oil pulling is based around the antibacterial properties of oil, which can kill the bacteria in the mouth that cause a host of issues such as cavities, plaque, and bad breath. The stain-removing power of baking soda and the minty freshness of peppermint essential oil create a superb toothpaste that is still gentle enough for use several times a day.

¼ cup coconut oil, soft but not melted

½ cup baking soda

1 teaspoon sea salt

15 drops peppermint essential oil

1. In a small bowl, stir together the coconut oil, baking soda, salt, and peppermint oil until it forms a paste.

2. Transfer the toothpaste to a glass container with a lid.

3. Store for up to 1 month at room temperature.

TIP Wet your toothbrush in clean water and scoop a dab of toothpaste onto the brush. Brush your teeth as suggested by your dentist and rinse out your mouth with clean water to finish. Make sure you also rinse your toothbrush thoroughly to remove any remaining toothpaste. A dirty toothbrush can harbor many types of damaging bacteria.

SUGAR LIP SCRUB

MAKES 3 TABLESPOONS • PREP TIME: 5 MINUTES • COOK TIME: 0 MINUTES

Soft pouty lips are only a sweet lip scrub away! Lips are an often-overlooked area of the body that can benefit from exfoliation as much as any other part of the skin. Scrubbing your lips will reduce chapped dry areas and minimize fine lines around the mouth. The bright scent of tangerine is pleasant, and this essential oil increases circulation so your lips stay plump and full.

1½ tablespoons coconut oil, melted

1 tablespoon coarse brown sugar

1 teaspoon honey

7 drops tangerine essential oil

1. Put the coconut oil, brown sugar, honey, and tangerine essential oil in a small bowl and stir to combine well.

2. Transfer the mixture to a jar with a lid.

3. Store the scrub at room temperature for up to 1 month.

TIP The skin on your lips is very delicate, so take care when using this scrub, especially if your lips are cracked at the corners or extremely chapped. Dip into the container with two fingertips and use small circular motions to buff your lips, starting with the top lip and working your way to the bottom. Use warm water to wash the scrub off after you are done exfoliating and finish with a soothing lip balm.

HOMEMADE LIP BALM

MAKES ¼ CUP • PREP TIME: 5 MINUTES • COOK TIME: 1 MINUTE

If you live in more extreme weather areas, you probably use lip balm extensively just to get through the seasons. This practice is necessary but can get expensive. Homemade lip balm is simple, and you can create different scents by changing the essential oil in the recipe. You have to make sure you choose oils that are nontoxic for your lip balms, such as rose, lavender, sweet orange, vanilla, and lemon.

3 tablespoons coconut oil

2 tablespoons beeswax

1 tablespoon shea butter

3 drops peppermint extract

1. Set a small saucepan over low heat and add the coconut oil, beeswax, and shea butter.

2. Stir the mixture until melted and well combined, about 1 minute.

3. Remove the saucepan from the heat, and stir in the peppermint extract.

4. Spoon the mixture into small glass containers with lids and let the lip balm harden.

5. Store the balm in the refrigerator for up to 3 months.

TIP Tiny jars and containers with lids can be found at any craft store for your lip balm needs. If you want to save some money, you can also use old lip balm tubes from purchased products that you might have hanging around in a drawer or makeup case. Simply wash the tube out thoroughly with soap and boiling water and refill the dry tubes with your own creations.

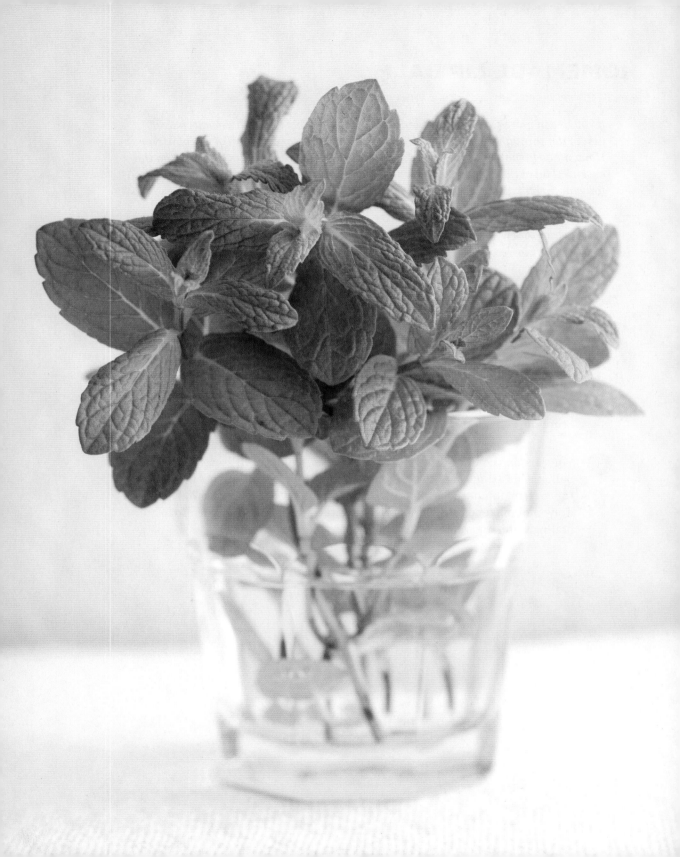

Chapter Five

THERAPEUTIC TREATMENTS

HOMEMADE VAPOR RUB

MAKES ¾ CUP • PREP TIME: 10 MINUTES • COOK TIME: 1 MINUTE

The menthol fragrance of the eucalyptus in this balm might take you back to your childhood, when Vicks VapoRub was a staple cure for coughs and stuffy noses. This homemade version of the familiar vapor rub is just as effective but without the sticky consistency. Rich with coconut oil and beeswax, it moisturizes the skin while the essential oils help ease breathing and clear a stuffed nose.

½ cup coconut oil

2 tablespoons beeswax

30 drops eucalyptus essential oil

10 drops lemon essential oil

10 drops peppermint essential oil

1. Set a small saucepan of water over medium-low heat and place a small bowl on the top of the saucepan so that the bottom is just above the water. Bring the water to a gentle simmer and reduce the heat to low.

2. Add the coconut oil and beeswax to the bowl and stir until melted and well combined, about 1 minute.

3. Remove the bowl from the top of the saucepan and add the eucalyptus, lemon, and peppermint essential oils. Stir to combine.

4. Spoon the mixture into a glass container with a lid and let the balm solidify.

5. Store the rub at room temperature for up to 6 months.

TIP This balm should not be used on children younger than eight years old, because peppermint and eucalyptus contain chemical constituents that are considered unsafe for that age range. To relieve chest or nasal congestion, rub a generous dab of this balm on your chest, breathing deeply to inhale the powerful essential oils. However, you don't have to wait till you have a cold to use this balm. For a good night's sleep, put a dab on your feet, rub it in, and go to bed with your coziest pair of socks on.

STIMULATING SCALP OIL

MAKES ½ CUP • PREP TIME: 3 MINUTES • COOK TIME: 0 MINUTES

The scalp needs moisture and nourishment in order to produce healthy, lush hair. If you ignore your scalp, you might experience hair loss and unsightly dandruff. Coconut oil is a wonderful base for any scalp treatment because it is moisturizing and can help reduce the inflammation that can stall hair growth. Rosemary essential oil can treat flaky dry scalp and help promote hair growth by stimulating the hair follicles and improving the thickness of the shaft.

½ cup coconut oil, softened but not melted

4 drops chamomile essential oil

4 drops rosemary essential oil

4 drops ylang ylang essential oil

1. In a small bowl, stir together the coconut oil and the chamomile, rosemary, and ylang ylang essential oils.

2. Transfer the mixture to a glass container with a lid.

3. Store the scalp oil at room temperature for up to 6 months.

TIP Before using the scalp oil, begin by brushing your hair with long strokes across your scalp to stimulate blood circulation and release any dry skin. Part your hair in the middle and apply the treatment with a cotton ball along the part. Continue parting your hair and dabbing your scalp in 1-inch sections all over your head. Then use your fingertips to massage the scalp in circular motions for about 20 minutes. Shampoo and condition as usual.

COCONUT COLD SORE RELIEF

MAKES 2 TABLESPOONS • PREP TIME: 5 MINUTES • COOK TIME: 2 MINUTES

Cold sores are incredibly painful and seem to appear at the most inopportune times, often triggered by stress and lack of sleep. Essential oils are quite effective for helping prevent breakouts and quickly healing the sores. Geranium oil can cut days off your healing time, and tea tree oil can help stop a cold sore from scabbing. The vitamin E in this balm can relieve the pain and scarring associated with the sores. Plus, the antiviral, antibiotic, and antifungal properties found in coconut oil help stop the spread of the virus that causes cold sores.

---

1 tablespoon coconut oil

1 tablespoon beeswax

¼ teaspoon vitamin E oil

7 drops peppermint essential oil

7 drops tea tree essential oil

6 drops lavender essential oil

5 drops geranium essential oil

1. Set a small saucepan of water over medium-low heat and place a small bowl on the top of the saucepan so that the bottom is just above the water. Bring the water to a gentle simmer and reduce the heat to low.

2. Add the coconut oil and beeswax to the bowl and stir until it is melted, about 2 minutes.

3. Remove the bowl from the top of the saucepan and stir in the vitamin E oil and the peppermint, tea tree, lavender, and geranium essential oils until the mixture is smooth and well blended.

4. Spoon the mixture into a glass container and let it cool completely.

5. Store for up to 6 months in a cool place.

TIP Apply the cold sore balm three to four times per day, beginning as soon as you feel the telltale tingle in your usual cold sore spot. If you get cold sores very close to the middle of your lips, it might be best to exclude the tea tree oil from this recipe, as this oil is extremely toxic when ingested.

SOOTHING HEADACHE BALM

MAKES ½ CUP • PREP TIME: 5 MINUTES • COOK TIME: 2 MINUTES

Headaches are caused by many different factors, and this recipe can be adjusted depending on what is causing your head to throb. The combination of essential oils in this base remedy is designed to alleviate a headache whose cause is unknown. If you know your headaches are stress related, then increase the lavender essential oil. If you get congestion-triggered headaches, then peppermint and eucalyptus should be increased by a few drops. Migraine headaches can often be affected positively by the addition of basil essential oil.

¼ cup coconut oil

2 tablespoons shea butter

10 drops peppermint oil

8 drops lavender essential oil

8 drops tea tree essential oil

4 drops eucalyptus essential oil

1. Set a small saucepan of water over medium-low heat and place a small bowl on the top of the saucepan so that the bottom is just above the water. Bring the water to a gentle simmer and reduce the heat to low.

2. Add the coconut oil and shea butter to the bowl and stir until it is melted, about 2 minutes.

3. Remove the bowl from the top of the saucepan and stir in the peppermint oil, and the lavender, tea tree, and eucalyptus essential oils until the mixture is smooth.

4. Spoon the mixture into a glass container with a lid, and let it cool completely until hardened, about 1 hour.

5. Store in a cool place so the balm stays hard, or in the refrigerator.

TIP   A little of this balm goes a long way, so only scoop out a tiny amount and rub it gently in a circular pattern on your temples, the back of your neck, and the skin above your sinuses. A gentle temple massage can also help reduce your headache pain when using this balm.

THERAPEUTIC TREATMENTS

LEMON-HONEY COUGH DROPS

MAKES ¾ CUP, OR ABOUT 24 DROPS • PREP TIME: 10 MINUTES • COOK TIME: 10 MINUTES

Cough drops are really just hard candies that have medicinal qualities rather than just calories and sugar. A sore throat and cough can be caused by many different factors, including bacteria and viruses. Honey makes a great base for these comforting morsels because it has antibacterial properties and a soothing consistency. Coconut oil is also an antibacterial and can help boost your immunity while you are fighting off a cold.

1 cup honey

3 tablespoons coconut oil

2 tablespoons lemon juice

5 drops therapeutic grade peppermint essential oil

Coconut oil for greasing a baking sheet

1. Lightly grease a baking sheet with coconut oil and set aside.

2. Set a small pot over medium heat and add the honey, coconut oil, lemon juice, and peppermint essential oil.

3. Bring the mixture to a boil, stirring.

4. Reduce the heat to low so that the honey mixture simmers.

5. Simmer until the mixture reaches 300°F on a candy thermometer, about 10 minutes.

6. Pour the honey mixture onto the prepared baking sheet and spread it out very carefully using a spatula.

7. Let the mixture cool until you can touch it and it is still very pliable.

8. Working quickly, pull off pieces of the mixture and roll into small ovals or rounds.

9. Put the cough drops back on a clean section of the baking sheet and let them harden completely.

10. Store the cough drops in a sealed glass container in a cool place for up to 1 month.

TIP There are no chemical or engineered ingredients in these all-natural drops, so take one whenever your throat is bothering you. If you want to create more child-friendly cough drops, lay lollipop sticks on your parchment and pour the honey mixture in a small pool at one end of each stick. Let the honey mixture harden, and you will have throat-soothing suckers.

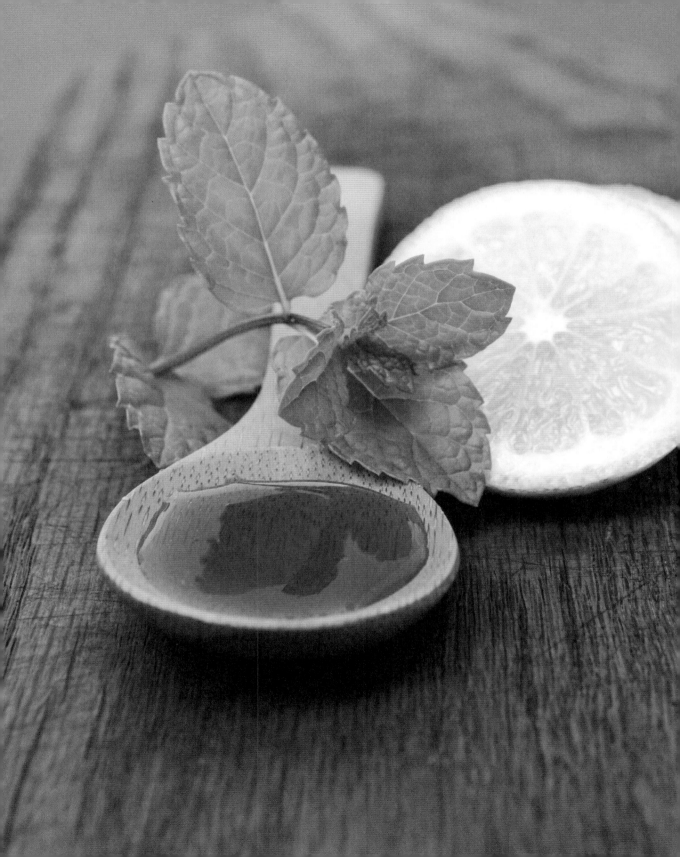

COCONUT OIL LICE TREATMENT

MAKES 1 TREATMENT • PREP TIME: 5 MINUTES • COOK TIME: 0 MINUTES

Just the idea of lice can make some people feel crawly. The standard treatments for lice often contain harsh chemicals and ingredients that can damage the scalp. This easy treatment takes about the same time as chemical treatments and contains only natural ingredients. The apple cider vinegar in this treatment will remove the lice eggs from the hair shafts. The coconut oil stops the lice from moving around, and the tea tree oil, a natural insecticide, will deliver the last, deadly blow.

1 to 2 cups coconut oil

10 drops tea tree essential oil

1 (15-ounce) bottle of apple cider vinegar

1. In a bowl, mix together the coconut oil and tea tree oils and set aside.

2. Completely rinse your hair top to bottom with the apple cider vinegar and let it dry on your hair.

3. When the vinegar is completely dry, coat your hair generously with the coconut oil mixture and massage it into the scalp.

4. Cover your head with a cap or towel and let the mixture sit for 12 hours on your head.

5. Comb your hair in sections with a fine-tooth comb to remove the dead lice and eggs.

6. Shampoo your hair thoroughly to remove the remaining oil.

TIP The amount of coconut oil and apple cider vinegar needed will depend entirely on the thickness and length of the hair involved in the infestation. Do not be stingy when applying either ingredient because the quicker you can get rid of the lice, the better.

PAIN-RELIEVING LOTION BAR

MAKES ¾ CUP OR 1 BAR • PREP TIME: 5 MINUTES, PLUS CHILLING TIME • COOK TIME: 2 MINUTES

Sore muscles and arthritis pain can be debilitating, so having a treatment on hand to provide quick relief is important. Coconut oil and shea butter melt luxuriously into the skin on contact and provide the perfect medium to transport pain-relieving frankincense essential oil to the joints. Studies done at Cardiff University have shown that frankincense oil inhibits the creation of cartilage-eroding molecules that eventually produce joint pain. The cedarwood and myrrh oils in this lotion also ease swollen and inflamed joints affected by arthritis.

¼ cup coconut oil

¼ cup beeswax

¼ cup shea butter

8 drops frankincense essential oil

8 drops lavender essential oil

4 drops cedarwood essential oil

4 drops myrrh essential oil

1. Set a small saucepan of water over medium-low heat and place a small bowl on the top of the saucepan so that the bottom is just above the water. Bring the water to a gentle simmer and reduce the heat to low.

2. Add the coconut oil, beeswax, and shea butter to the bowl and stir until it is melted, about 2 minutes.

3. Remove the bowl from the top of the saucepan and stir in the frankincense, lavender, cedarwood, and myrrh essential oils until the mixture is smooth.

4. Spoon the mixture into a bar-shaped mold (or an ice pop mold) and let it cool completely until hardened, about 1 hour.

5. Pop the bar out of the mold and store it in a sealed glass container in a cool place so the bar stays hard, or store it in the refrigerator.

6. You can store this remedy for up to 6 months.

TIP Take the bar out of the refrigerator and cut off as much as you need for the area that is sore. Melt the bar by rubbing your palms together, and apply the ointment to the affected area, massaging it deeply into the skin. You can use an ice pop mold to form the bar, or ice cube trays if you want to just take a smaller one out without cutting the bar.

HEALING BURN SALVE

MAKES ¾ CUP • PREP TIME: 10 MINUTES • COOK TIME: 4 MINUTES

Make sure to use raw, unpasteurized honey for this salve, as pasteurization can kill the phytonutrients that contribute to honey's antiseptic and antibacterial effects. Honey can stimulate the growth of new skin and prevent infection when applied to burned skin. The coconut oil and aloe vera are incredibly soothing and help repair the damaged areas quickly.

6 tablespoons coconut oil

2 teaspoons beeswax

¼ cup raw honey

1 tablespoon vitamin E oil

1 teaspoon aloe vera gel

8 drops lavender essential oil

1. Set a small saucepan of water over medium-low heat and place a small bowl on the top of the saucepan so that the bottom is just above the water. Bring the water to a gentle simmer and reduce the heat to low.

2. Add the coconut oil and beeswax to the bowl and stir until it is melted, about 4 minutes.

3. Remove the bowl from the top of the saucepan and stir in the honey, vitamin E oil, aloe vera gel, and lavender essential oil until the mixture is smooth and well blended.

4. Spoon the mixture into a glass container and let it cool completely for about 1 hour before putting on the lid. Let the balm harden completely before using.

5. Store the salve for up to 6 months in either a cool place or the refrigerator.

TIP Use this salve immediately after the burn happens and continue applying it until the injury is healed. This salve is not meant for serious burns that require medical attention.

CUT & SCRAPE CREAM

MAKES 1¼ CUPS • PREP TIME: 10 MINUTES • COOK TIME: 4 MINUTES

If you have kids in your home, there is a very good chance that someone has a cut, scrape, or bruise at any given moment. Coconut oil and honey will help fight any infection-causing bacteria, giving the skin a chance to heal cleanly and quickly. Almond oil is packed with antioxidants that reduce the risk of inflammation and help new skin grow. Lavender oil is a safe antibacterial to use with children, and the fragrance can help calm a teary patient when the upset is worse than the actual injury.

½ cup coconut oil

½ cup sweet almond oil

¼ cup beeswax

1 tablespoon honey

10 drops chamomile essential oil

10 drops lavender essential oil

7 drops tea tree essential oil

1. Set a small saucepan of water over medium-low heat and place a small bowl on the top of the saucepan so that the bottom is just above the water. Bring the water to a gentle simmer and reduce the heat to low.

2. Add the coconut oil, sweet almond oil, and beeswax to the bowl and stir until it is melted, about 4 minutes.

3. Remove the bowl from the top of the saucepan and stir in the honey and the chamomile, lavender, and tea tree essential oils until the mixture is smooth and well blended.

4. Spoon the mixture into a glass container and let it cool completely, stirring occasionally.

5. Store the cream for up to 6 months in a cool place.

TIP   Spread this cream generously over small cuts and scrapes after cleaning the area thoroughly. You can apply a bandage over the cream if the cut warrants extra protection. This balm is not meant to be used on serious cuts that require medical attention.

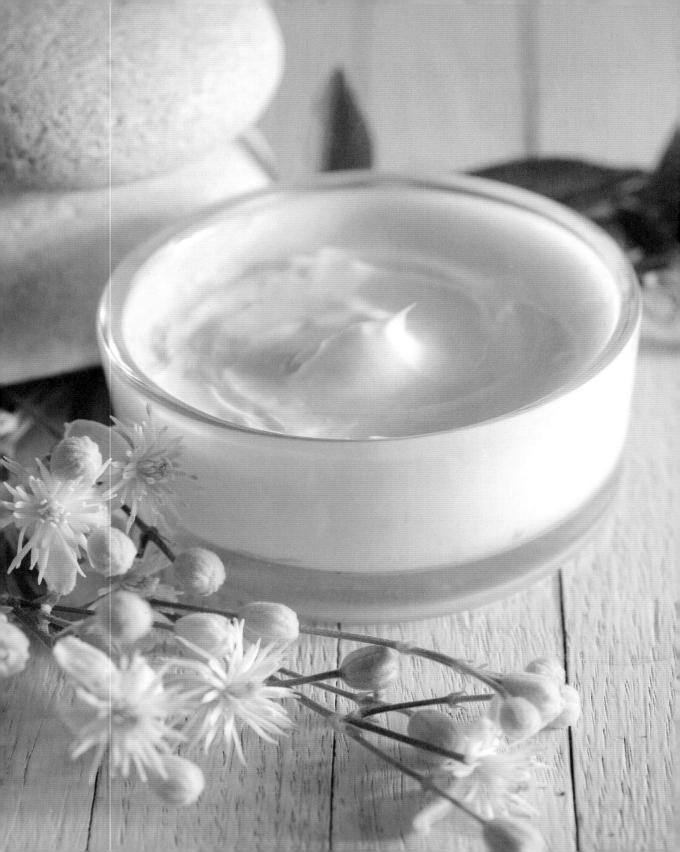

SLEEPY-TIME BALM

MAKES 1½ CUPS • PREP TIME: 15 MINUTES PLUS CHILLING TIME • COOK TIME: 2 MINUTES

Lavender is probably the best known natural remedy for insomnia and anxiety, so it is featured in this whipped, fragrant balm. A study in the United Kingdom concluded that 20 percent of people who use lavender experience a better sleep than those who do not. Roman chamomile is often combined with lavender for sleep-related issues and has been used for centuries. It is important to omit the chamomile in this recipe if you are pregnant, because it can cause uterine contractions. The neroli oil or orange blossom oil is a treatment for hypertension and stress—it will help you let go of the anxiety that can make sleep difficult.

½ cup coconut oil

½ cup cocoa butter

15 drops lavender essential oil

10 drops Roman chamomile essential oil

5 drops neroli essential oil

5 drops rosewood essential oil

1. Set a small saucepan over low heat and add the coconut oil and cocoa butter.

2. Stir until melted and well combined, about 2 minutes.

3. Transfer the coconut oil mixture to a medium stainless steel bowl and stir in the lavender, Roman chamomile, neroli, and rosewood essential oils until well blended, about 30 seconds.

4. Put the bowl in the refrigerator until the mixture is starting to solidify but is not completely solid, about 15 to 20 minutes.

5. Use an electric hand beater to whip the mixture until it is very light and fluffy, about 10 minutes, scraping down the sides of the bowl at least once.

6. Spoon the whipped mixture into a glass jar with a lid and store at room temperature for up to 2 months.

TIP Take a small amount, about the size of a pencil eraser, and massage it into your feet or your children's feet before bed. Cover with comfy socks and drift off to sleep.

COCONUT ECZEMA CREAM

MAKES ½ CUP • PREP TIME: 5 MINUTES • COOK TIME: 0 MINUTES

The shea butter and coconut oil that form the base of this healing cream penetrate deeply into the skin and provide relief from the itchiness associated with eczema. These ingredients, along with vitamin E, can reduce the inflammation that is thought to be a key contributor to flare-ups of this painful skin condition. Lavender is also an anti-inflammatory, and it contains natural antiseptic properties that can help soothe pain and itchy skin.

¼ cup coconut oil, melted

3 tablespoons shea butter

½ teaspoon vitamin E oil

15 drops lavender essential oil

10 drops tea tree essential oil

5 drops clove essential oil

5 drops rosemary essential oil

1. In a small bowl, stir together the coconut oil, shea butter, and vitamin E oil until blended, about 2 minutes.

2. Add in the lavender, tea tree, clove, and rosemary essential oils and stir to blend.

3. Spoon the mixture into a glass container with a lid and store in a cool place or in the refrigerator so that it remains hardened.

4. You can store this cream for up to 6 months.

TIP   Smooth this cream on all your affected areas and gently massage it into the skin. The texture will prevent you from applying too much, but if you have large areas of dry skin to treat, you can let it sit in a warm spot to soften for easier application.

SOFT BABY-BOTTOM CREAM

MAKES ¾ CUP • PREP TIME: 20 MINUTES PLUS CHILLING TIME • COOK TIME: 4 MINUTES

The delicate, petal-smooth skin on your baby's bottom needs to be protected to eliminate the risk of painful diaper rash and chafing. Lavender and chamomile essential oils are perfect choices for a cream to apply topically, because they are considered safe for use on infants over the age of three months. The beeswax is an effective barrier for any wetness that occurs after the application of the balm, and the shea butter can heal an existing rash.

---

6 tablespoons coconut oil

5 tablespoons shea butter

4 tablespoons beeswax

4 drops chamomile essential oil

4 drops lavender essential oil

1. Set a small saucepan over low heat and add the coconut oil, shea butter, and beeswax.

2. Stir until melted and well combined, about 4 minutes.

3. Transfer the coconut oil mixture to a medium stainless steel bowl and stir in the chamomile and lavender essential oils until well blended, about 30 seconds.

4. Put the bowl in the refrigerator until the mixture is starting to solidify but is not completely solid, about 15 to 20 minutes.

5. Use an electric hand beater on medium speed to whip the mixture until it is very light and fluffy, about 10 minutes, scraping down the sides of the bowl at least once.

6. Put a glass jar big enough to hold 2 cups of balm and the lid in a pot of boiling water for 10 minutes to sterilize. Set the jar on a cooling rack to dry.

7. Spoon the body butter into the glass jar and store at room temperature for up to 2 months.

TIP Do not use any essential oil product on infants younger than three months, because their skin is much more permeable than that of adults. This cream is still effective for preventing diaper rash without the essential oils, so omit them until your child reaches three months old.

FLORAL ANTI-INFLAMMATORY CREAM

MAKES 1 CUP • PREP TIME: 10 MINUTES • COOK TIME: 4 MINUTES

Skin inflammation can cause severe discomfort, and finding relief can be frustrating and expensive. Every ingredient in this cream helps fight inflammation, and you will be delighted by the spring garden scent. Olive oil is packed with antioxidants, including a compound called oleocanthal that blocks an enzyme responsible for skin inflammation. German chamomile contains a natural chemical called azulene, which is a very powerful anti-inflammatory. And calendula can significantly reduce inflammation and speed healing.

½ cup coconut oil

2 tablespoons olive oil

1 tablespoon beeswax

10 drops German chamomile essential oil

10 drops lavender essential oil

6 drops calendula essential oil

1. Set a small saucepan of water over medium-low heat and place a small bowl on the top of the saucepan so that the bottom is just above the water. Bring the water to a gentle simmer and reduce the heat to low.

2. Add the coconut oil, olive oil, and beeswax to the bowl and stir until it is melted, about 4 minutes.

3. Remove the bowl from the top of the saucepan and stir in the German chamomile, lavender, and calendula essential oils until the mixture is smooth and well blended.

4. Spoon the mixture into a glass container and let it cool completely.

5. Store the cream for up to 6 months in a cool place.

TIP Smooth this cream on inflamed skin and bruises to speed up the healing process and eliminate redness and pain.

BUGS-BE-GONE BALM

MAKES 1 CUP • PREP TIME: 10 MINUTES • COOK TIME: 4 MINUTES

Nothing ruins an outdoor adventure faster than swarms of mosquitos and blackflies teeming around your family. There are many essential oils that are extremely effective against bugs, and the combination in this recipe works on many common pests. Mosquitos can be repelled with all the oils used in this balm. Fleas and ticks will stay away from cedarwood, citronella, lavender, lemongrass, and peppermint. Horseflies steer clear of lavender, lemongrass, peppermint, and rosemary.

¾ cup coconut oil

¼ cup shea butter

3 tablespoons beeswax

20 drops citronella essential oil

10 drops cedarwood essential oil

10 drops lavender essential oil

10 drops lemongrass essential oil

10 drops peppermint essential oil

10 drops rosemary essential oil

1. Set a small saucepan of water over medium-low heat and place a small bowl on the top of the saucepan so that the bottom is just above the water. Bring the water to a gentle simmer and reduce the heat to low.

2. Add the coconut oil, shea butter, and beeswax to the bowl and stir until it is melted, about 4 minutes.

3. Remove the bowl from the top of the saucepan and stir in the essential oils until the mixture is smooth and well blended.

4. Spoon the mixture into a glass container and let it cool completely before putting on the lid, about 1 hour.

5. Store the balm at room temperature for up to 3 months.

TIP Apply this balm lightly to all exposed skin except the face at least 30 minutes before going outside, and reapply if you are swimming or sweating profusely in the heat. This cream contains a potent concentration of essential oils, and it should not be used on pregnant women or children younger than eight years old.

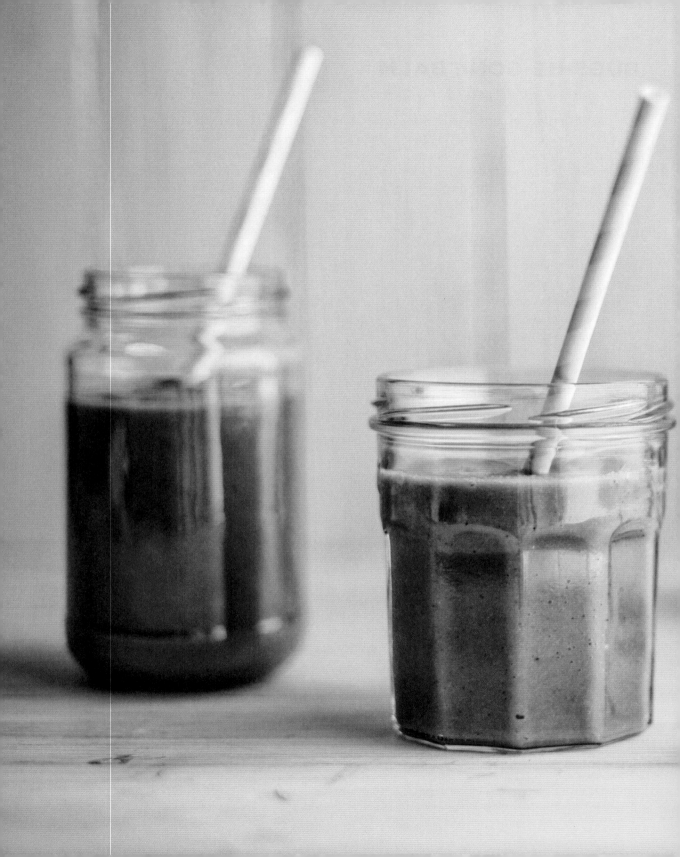

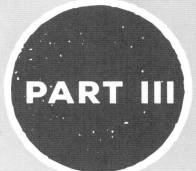

PART III

Food & Drink

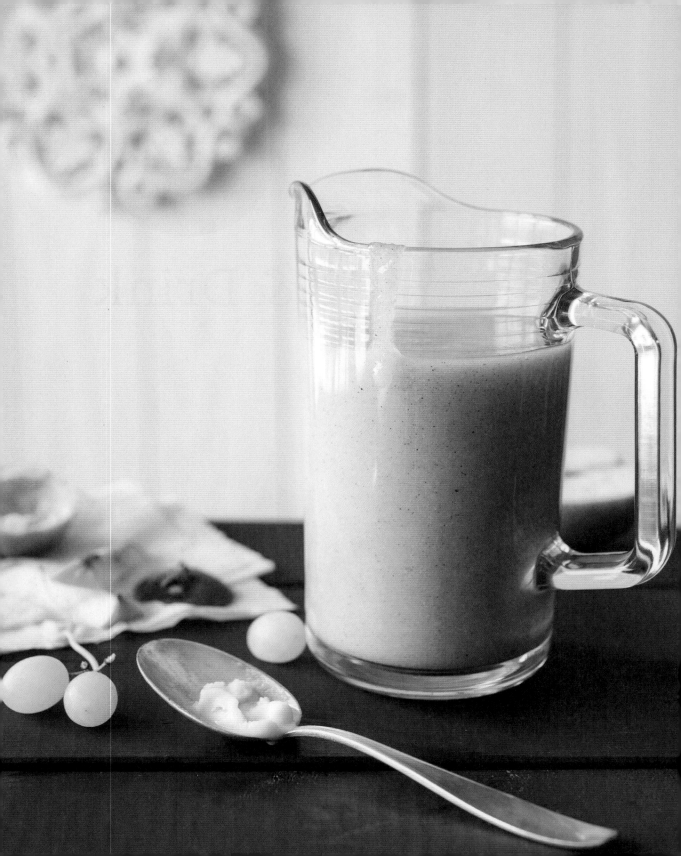

Chapter Six

DRINKS & SMOOTHIES

HOMEMADE COCONUT MILK

PALEO-FRIENDLY VEGAN GLUTEN-FREE

MAKES 4 CUPS • PREP TIME: 15 MINUTES • COOK TIME: 5 MINUTES

This recipe does not make the rich, thick coconut milk you get in cans but rather the thinner product in cartons in the dairy section. Store-bought coconut milk can get quite expensive if you want to use it extensively in your recipes, so it might be a good idea to make your own. The taste and texture of homemade milk is almost identical to packaged coconut milk, and you still get all the antibacterial, antiviral, and antifungal properties.

4 cups filtered water   2 cups shredded unsweetened coconut

1. Pour the water into a large saucepan over medium-high heat. Heat the water until it is very hot but not boiling, about 5 minutes.

2. Add the coconut and hot water to a blender and process on high until the mixture is creamy, about 4 minutes.

3. Pour the liquid through a fine-mesh sieve to remove the majority of the shredded coconut.

4. Pour the strained liquid through a double layer of fine cheesecloth to catch the remaining coconut. Squeeze the solid bits in the cloth to get all the liquid.

5. Store the coconut milk in a sealed container in the refrigerator for 3 to 4 days.

6. Shake the coconut milk before each use.

TIP   After you squeeze out every drop of coconut milk from the cheesecloth, the solids left in the cheesecloth can be used as coconut flour. Spread the contents on a baking sheet and let them dry completely, stirring occasionally. Then return the pulverized coconut to a food processor and purée until very finely chopped.

COCONUT CHOCOLATE MILK

PALEO-FRIENDLY GLUTEN-FREE

SERVES 2 • PREP TIME: 5 MINUTES • COOK TIME: 0 MINUTES

If you are a fan of chocolate milk, this coconut version will become your new favorite. The richness of the coconut milk and coconut oil combines beautifully with cocoa to create a beverage that tastes like liquid chocolate. Try to find Dutch-process cocoa powder rather than natural cocoa because the Dutch product is washed with a potassium solution, which neutralizes the acidity, darkens the color, and creates a mellow, pleasing flavor.

---

3 cups canned light coconut milk

½ cup almonds

¼ cup cocoa powder

¼ cup honey

¼ cup coconut oil

1 teaspoon pure vanilla extract

Pinch ground cinnamon

1. Put the coconut milk, almonds, cocoa powder, honey, coconut oil, vanilla, and cinnamon in a blender and blend until smooth.

2. Pour into 2 glasses and serve immediately.

TIP There are more than 700 compounds in cocoa, including powerful antioxidants such as polyphenols, which promote cardiovascular health. Polyphenols protect the cardiovascular system by lowering bad cholesterol and reducing the risk of arteriosclerosis.

LEMON COCONUT MILKSHAKE

PALEO-FRIENDLY GLUTEN-FREE

SERVES 2 • PREP TIME: 5 MINUTES • COOK TIME: 0 MINUTES

The frozen banana in this smoothie gives it the creamy, thick milkshake texture, so if you only have a fresh banana, throw in a couple of ice cubes with the rest of the ingredients. It's best to peel a banana before freezing it; however, if you leave the peel on, don't let the dark frozen skin concern you—the banana remains sweet and perfect for a smoothie.

---

2 cups canned light coconut milk

1 frozen banana

¼ cup freshly squeezed lemon juice

3 tablespoons coconut oil

1 tablespoon honey

2 teaspoons lemon zest

2 teaspoons pure vanilla extract

1. Put the coconut milk, banana, lemon juice, coconut oil, honey, lemon zest, and vanilla in a blender and blend until smooth.

2. Pour into 2 glasses and serve immediately.

BANANA YOGURT DRINK

GLUTEN-FREE

SERVES 2 • PREP TIME: 5 MINUTES • COOK TIME: 0 MINUTES

Try this sweet, tangy beverage plain or with a sprinkling of toasted coconut for a special treat. You can double up on the banana flavor by using banana yogurt instead of plain or another flavor for an interesting variation. If you want your smoothie to be vegan, swap in coconut or soy yogurt instead of regular cow's milk yogurt.

---

1 cup canned light coconut milk

1 cup plain yogurt

2 bananas

2 tablespoons coconut oil

4 almonds

6 ice cubes

1. Put the coconut milk, yogurt, bananas, coconut oil, almonds, and ice cubes in a blender and blend until smooth.

2. Pour into 2 glasses and serve immediately.

RASPBERRY YOGURT SMOOTHIE

GLUTEN-FREE

SERVES 2 • PREP TIME: 5 MINUTES • COOK TIME: 0 MINUTES

You might think you are drinking a berry cheesecake when you first try this smoothie, even with the crunch of raspberry seeds. Greek yogurt is tangy and packed with protein because the whey has been strained out to create a thick, creamy product. You can use plain regular yogurt instead, but the texture will not be as rich and dense.

---

1 cup plain Greek yogurt

1 cup frozen raspberries

1 cup shredded unsweetened coconut

½ cup canned light coconut milk

¼ teaspoon ground cinnamon

1. Put the yogurt, raspberries, coconut, coconut milk, and cinnamon in a blender and blend until smooth.

2. Pour into 2 glasses and serve immediately.

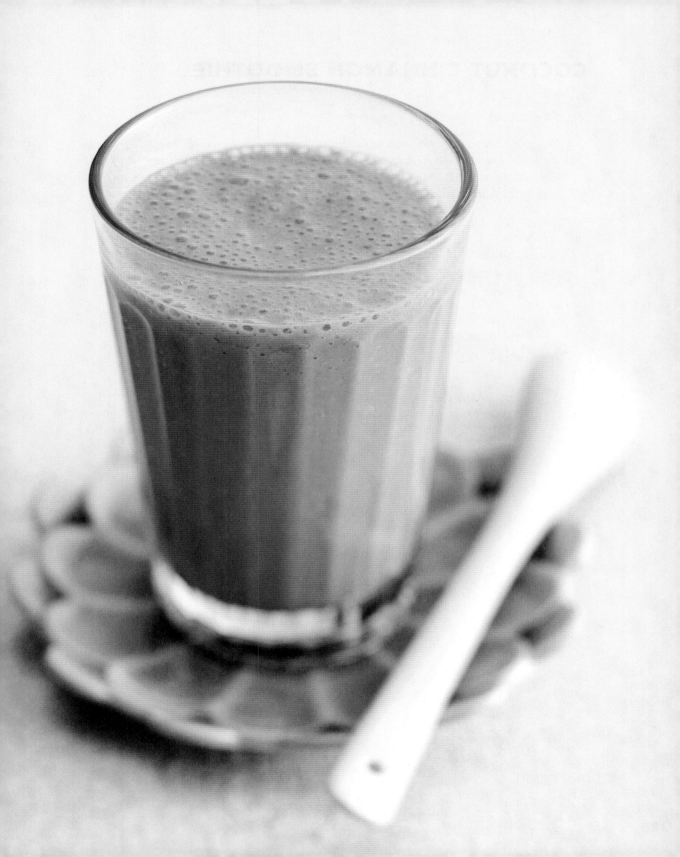

COCONUT-CINNAMON SMOOTHIE

GLUTEN-FREE

SERVES 2 • PREP TIME: 5 MINUTES • COOK TIME: 0 MINUTES

Cinnamon is used extensively in many cuisines across the world, which is probably why most people find its scent familiar and comforting. This warm spice is a good source of fiber and is high in calcium and manganese, which can help reduce cholesterol levels and regulate blood sugar.

---

3 cups milk

2 frozen bananas

¼ cup shredded unsweetened coconut

1 tablespoon coconut oil

1 teaspoon pure vanilla extract

¼ teaspoon cinnamon

1. Put the milk, bananas, coconut, coconut oil, vanilla, and cinnamon in a blender and blend until smooth.

2. Pour into 2 glasses and serve immediately.

TIP Some of the cinnamon you see in the grocery store is not technically cinnamon, from the bark of the cinnamon tree, but actually cassia cinnamon, which comes from a different plant. True cinnamon, or Ceylon cinnamon, has extraordinary health benefits and a delicately sweet flavor. Cassia is pungent and strong and has a high level of coumarin, which acts as a powerful blood thinner and can be damaging to the liver. Try to find Ceylon cinnamon for your recipes.

GREEN COCONUT SMOOTHIE

PALEO-FRIENDLY GLUTEN-FREE

SERVES 2 • PREP TIME: 5 MINUTES • COOK TIME: 0 MINUTES

There are many different coconut waters flooding the market these days, making it hard to determine the best product to buy. Less-processed coconut water has the most nutrients, so stay away from concentrated products that have been produced from syrup. Try to get unpasteurized coconut water from young coconuts with no added sweeteners.

2 cups coconut water

2 kiwifruits, peeled

1 cup green grapes

1 green apple, cored

2 tablespoons coconut oil

1 tablespoon honey

1. Put the coconut water, kiwifruits, grapes, apple, coconut oil, and honey in a blender and blend until smooth.

2. Pour into 2 glasses and serve immediately.

BLUEBERRY-VANILLA-COCONUT SMOOTHIE

PALEO-FRIENDLY VEGAN GLUTEN-FREE

SERVES 2 • PREP TIME: 5 MINUTES • COOK TIME: 0 MINUTES

Smoothies are meant to replace a meal, usually breakfast, so recipes sometimes contain ingredients that seem out of place in what seems like a tasty milkshake. Since the idea is to pack as much nutrition into one glass, 1 tablespoon of flaxseed is a logical choice. Flaxseed is a superb source of omega-3 essential fatty acids and fiber. This means that the toasty, tasty seed can cut the risk of diabetes, cancer, and heart disease.

---

2 cups almond milk

2 cups blueberries

½ cup shredded unsweetened coconut

2 tablespoons coconut oil

1 tablespoon flaxseed

2 teaspoons pure vanilla extract

6 ice cubes

1. Put the almond milk, blueberries, coconut, coconut oil, flaxseed, vanilla, and ice cubes in a blender and blend until smooth.

2. Pour into 2 glasses and serve immediately.

COCONUT PROTEIN SMOOTHIE

VEGAN

SERVES 2 • PREP TIME: 5 MINUTES • COOK TIME: 0 MINUTES

This smoothie is just the thing your body needs after an intense workout. Protein helps to replenish your body's nutrients and aid in muscle recovery, and coconut oil can replenish a fatty acid (intramuscular fatty acid) that boosts cell growth and provides energy for muscle cells. You can also try this protein smoothie for an afternoon energy boost on a busy day.

---

2 cups canned light coconut milk

2 frozen bananas

⅓ cup vegan protein powder

¼ cup oat flakes

2 tablespoons coconut oil, melted

2 teaspoons pure vanilla extract

¼ teaspoon ground cinnamon

1. Put the coconut milk, bananas, protein powder, oat flakes, coconut oil, vanilla, and cinnamon in a blender and blend until smooth.

2. Pour into 2 glasses and serve immediately.

BANANA-COCONUT-CHIA SMOOTHIE

VEGAN GLUTEN-FREE

SERVES 2 • PREP TIME: 5 MINUTES • COOK TIME: 0 MINUTES

Bananas are a popular ingredient in smoothies because they add thickness and a delicious sweetness that can mask the flavor of less palatable ingredients. If you want a very tropical smoothie, replace 1 banana with 1 cup of fresh pineapple, and top the drink with a scattering of toasted coconut.

---

2 cups canned light coconut milk

1 tablespoon chia seeds

2 bananas

2 tablespoons coconut oil

Pinch ground nutmeg

1. Combine the coconut milk and chia seeds in a medium bowl, then cover the bowl and refrigerate overnight.

2. Pour the coconut milk mixture into a blender along with the bananas, coconut oil, and nutmeg and blend until smooth.

3. Pour into 2 glasses and serve immediately.

TIP This smoothie is a plan-ahead drink because you have to soak the chia seeds before using them, or the smoothie will be gritty and not as thick. When you take the bowl out of the refrigerator in the morning, do not be surprised by the pudding-like consistency of the chia mixture. Chia seeds can soak up about nine times their weight of liquid.

PAPAYA-COCONUT SMOOTHIE

PALEO-FRIENDLY VEGAN GLUTEN-FREE

SERVES 2 • PREP TIME: 5 MINUTES • COOK TIME: 0 MINUTES

Papaya is a lush, interesting-looking fruit with glorious deeply hued flesh and dark pearly seeds. This smoothie is a little thinner in texture, but the color is like a sunset. If you want a thicker smoothie, substitute coconut milk for the coconut water, or add 3 or 4 ice cubes to your blender. Make sure your papaya is ripe, with an almost buttery texture, to get the best taste.

2 cups coconut water

2 cups chopped papaya flesh

1 banana

2 tablespoons coconut oil

1. Put the coconut water, papaya, banana, and coconut oil in a blender and blend until smooth.

2. Pour into 2 glasses and serve immediately.

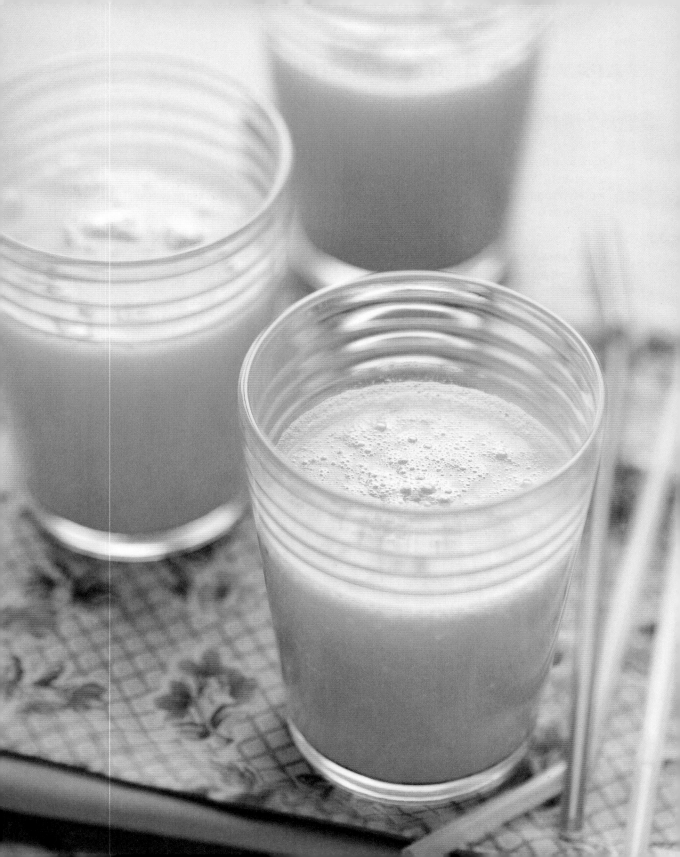

COCONUT-PEACH SMOOTHIE

PALEO-FRIENDLY VEGAN GLUTEN-FREE

SERVES 2 • PREP TIME: 5 MINUTES • COOK TIME: 0 MINUTES

Peaches are so lush and fragrant you will feel decadent when enjoying this pretty pastel drink. You do not have to remove the fuzzy skin before chopping the fruit up, but make sure you wash the skin thoroughly, even if you purchase organic produce. This smoothie can be made with frozen peaches as well, but the flavor will not be as intense.

2 cups canned light coconut milk

2 cups chopped fresh peaches

1 banana

¼ cup shredded unsweetened coconut

1 tablespoon coconut oil

1. Put the coconut milk, peaches, banana, coconut, and coconut oil in a blender and blend until smooth.

2. Pour into 2 glasses and serve immediately.

KALE-MANGO SMOOTHIE

GLUTEN-FREE

SERVES 2 • PREP TIME: 5 MINUTES • COOK TIME: 0 MINUTES

Mango is a culinary delight that flaunts outrageous brightly hued flesh and a sweet taste. The mango combines well with the kale, especially if you use lacinato kale, which is earthy and slightly nutty rather than bitter like curly kale. If you can only find curly kale in your local store, try to get young, tender leaves for a milder flavor.

1 cup coconut water

2 cups chopped kale

½ cup plain yogurt

1 banana

1 mango, peeled, pitted, and chopped

1. Put the coconut water, kale, yogurt, banana, and mango in a blender and blend until smooth. Add more coconut water if you want a thinner texture.

2. Pour into 2 glasses and serve immediately.

COCONUT-PUMPKIN SMOOTHIE

PALEO-FRIENDLY GLUTEN-FREE

SERVES 2 • PREP TIME: 5 MINUTES • COOK TIME: 0 MINUTES

Creamy warm spiced pumpkin pie in a glass. The color and flavor of this smoothie are so exceptional that you will want to make this recipe more than once. Transfer the extra canned pumpkin to an airtight container and keep it handy in the fridge for whenever another craving strikes. Pumpkin is an excellent source of beta-carotene, vitamins A and C, fiber, and potassium, so including it regularly in your diet will help flush toxins from your body and cut your risk of cancer.

---

2 cups canned coconut milk

2 bananas

½ cup pure pumpkin purée

2 tablespoons coconut oil

1 tablespoon honey

¼ teaspoon ground cinnamon

Pinch ground nutmeg

1. Put the coconut milk, bananas, pumpkin, coconut oil, honey, cinnamon, and nutmeg in a blender and blend until smooth.

2. Pour into 2 glasses and serve immediately.

TIP   Roasted mashed pumpkin can be substituted for canned pumpkin purée with impressive results. If you are using a canned product for convenience, avoid pie filling, which has extra sugar and spices that you do not need in your smoothie.

BEET-COCONUT SMOOTHIE

PALEO-FRIENDLY VEGAN GLUTEN-FREE

SERVES 2 • PREP TIME: 5 MINUTES • COOK TIME: 0 MINUTES

Beets become sweet and rich when they are cooked, adding a complex pleasing flavor and vibrant red color to this smoothie. When you combine this versatile vegetable with strawberries and pineapple, it might seem like you are drinking dessert. Tempt your kids with this rosy, almost sugary, drink when you want them to get a healthy dose of antioxidants and vitamins in the morning.

---

2 cups canned light coconut milk

2 cooked, peeled beets

1 cup pineapple

1 cup frozen strawberries

2 tablespoons coconut oil

Pinch ground nutmeg

1. Put the coconut milk, beets, pineapple, strawberries, coconut oil, and nutmeg in a blender and blend until smooth.

2. Pour into 2 glasses and serve immediately.

TIP If you want to further enhance the delicious taste of your beets, try roasting them instead of boiling them. The skin will not be as easy to remove, but the flavor is incredible.

GREEN TEA WITH COCONUT OIL

PALEO-FRIENDLY GLUTEN-FREE

SERVES 2 • PREP TIME: 1 MINUTE • COOK TIME: 3 MINUTES

It might seem very strange to add oil to a cup of tea or to any hot beverage such as coffee. You will not make the drink greasy as long as the amount of oil is not excessive. Drink the tea while it is still hot so the oil remains suspended in the liquid. You can omit the honey in this beverage and add agave nectar instead if you want a vegan drink.

---

1 tablespoon honey

2 tablespoons coconut oil

Juice of 1 lemon

2 green tea bags

Water heated to just boiling

Pinch ground nutmeg

1. Add the honey, coconut oil, and lemon juice to a teapot or divide the ingredients evenly between 2 cups. Stir to combine.

2. Add the tea bags and water to the pot or cups and let the tea steep for 3 minutes.

3. Remove the tea bags and add a pinch of nutmeg.

4. Stir to blend and serve immediately.

TIP
When drawing water to make tea, start with cold water rather than warm because cold water has more oxygen in it, which helps develop the flavor of the tea. When the water just starts to boil, it is ready for the tea, but do not allow the water to continue boiling before pouring it over the tea, or it can scald the leaves.

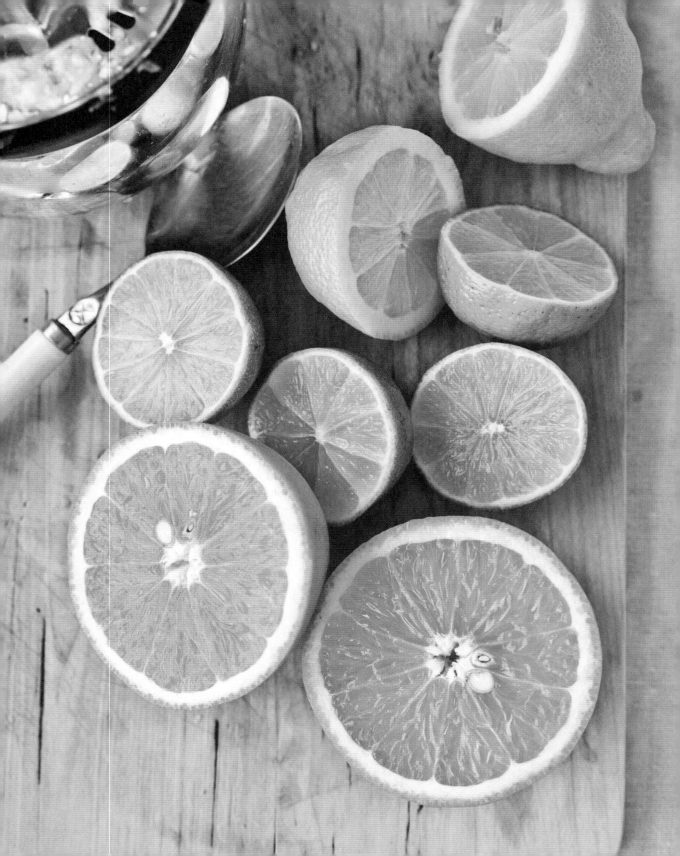

Chapter Seven

BREAKFAST

COCONUT-VANILLA CREAM WITH STRAWBERRIES

GLUTEN-FREE

SERVES 4 • PREP TIME: 10 MINUTES PLUS CHILLING TIME • COOK TIME: 10 MINUTES

Who says you can't have a creamy, luscious pudding topped with ripe berries for breakfast? Coconut milk creates a lovely silky textured pudding with a hint of nuttiness that is accented by the shredded coconut topping. You can use any fruit that you have handy, including peaches, other berries, cherries, or oranges.

2½ cups canned coconut milk

¼ cup granulated sugar

¼ cup arrowroot flour

1 egg

1 teaspoon coconut oil

2 teaspoons pure vanilla extract

2 cups sliced strawberries

¼ cup shredded sweetened coconut

1. In a medium saucepan over medium heat, whisk together the coconut milk, sugar, and arrowroot flour.

2. Bring the coconut milk mixture to a boil and then reduce the heat to low and continue whisking until the pudding is thick and creamy, about 4 minutes.

3. Whisk the egg into the pudding and continue to cook for about 30 seconds.

4. Whisk in the coconut oil and vanilla.

5. Remove the pudding from the heat and let it cool in the refrigerator with plastic wrap pressed to the surface of the pudding until completely chilled.

6. Serve topped with sliced strawberries and shredded coconut.

MAPLE RICE BREAKFAST PUDDING

VEGAN GLUTEN-FREE

SERVES 4 • PREP TIME: 5 MINUTES • COOK TIME: 30 MINUTES

Rice pudding is just another version of hot cereal, which can be a nice change from oatmeal or a cream of wheat product. Rice is a staple food for more than half the world's population, and this grain is grown in over 100 countries. Basmati rice originates in India and is characterized by a distinctive nutty aroma that combines very well with coconut. You can use brown basmati rice if you prefer a chewier texture.

---

1 cup basmati rice

1 (15-ounce) can full-fat coconut milk

1 teaspoon pure vanilla extract

Pinch sea salt

½ cup shredded unsweetened coconut

½ cup raisins

½ cup chopped pecans

¼ cup maple syrup

1. Put the rice, coconut milk, vanilla, and salt in a large saucepan and put it over medium heat.

2. Bring the rice to a boil and then reduce the heat to low, cover, and simmer until the rice is tender, stirring frequently, about 30 minutes.

3. Remove the saucepan from the heat and stir in the coconut, raisins, pecans, and maple syrup.

4. Adjust the texture of the recipe with milk if you want your cereal a little thinner.

5. Serve warm.

TIP You might not realize that there are grades of maple syrup with different appearance and flavors. The best choice for this recipe is Grade A Dark Amber or #3 Dark (D) if the syrup comes from Canada. Maple syrup can also be cut with high-fructose corn syrup, so make sure you get a 100 percent pure maple product, organic preferred.

DATE ENERGY BARS

PALEO-FRIENDLY **VEGAN** GLUTEN-FREE

MAKES 16 BARS • PREP TIME: 10 MINUTES PLUS CHILLING TIME • COOK TIME: 0 MINUTES

Store-bought energy bars often have ingredient lists that cover the entire label, and many of the listed items look like chemistry experiments. On the other hand, these bars are made of all-natural ingredients and will fuel you just as well, or better, than the store-bought ones. You can make a double batch of the bars and freeze a container full so that you always have a grab-and-go snack available.

---

1 cup shredded unsweetened coconut

1 cup dates

1 cup gluten-free oats

1 cup pumpkin seeds

½ cup dried blueberries

½ cup raisins

½ cup sesame seeds

2 tablespoons melted coconut oil

½ cup mini chocolate chips

1. Line a 9-by-13-inch baking dish with parchment and set aside.
2. Put the coconut, dates, oats, pumpkin seeds, blueberries, raisins, sesame seeds, and coconut oil in a food processor and pulse until everything sticks together but is still chunky.
3. If the mixture does not seem to hold together, add a little more coconut oil.
4. Dump the mixture into the baking dish and use your hands to incorporate the chocolate chips.
5. Press the coconut mixture into the baking dish evenly and put the dish in the refrigerator until the bars can be cut, about 2 hours.
6. Store the bars in a sealed container in the refrigerator for up to 1 week

TIP You can use date paste for this recipe instead of whole dates as long as the paste is 100 percent dates with no unnecessary fillers. When looking for whole dates, choose Medjool dates if they are available because this is the sweetest and largest variety.

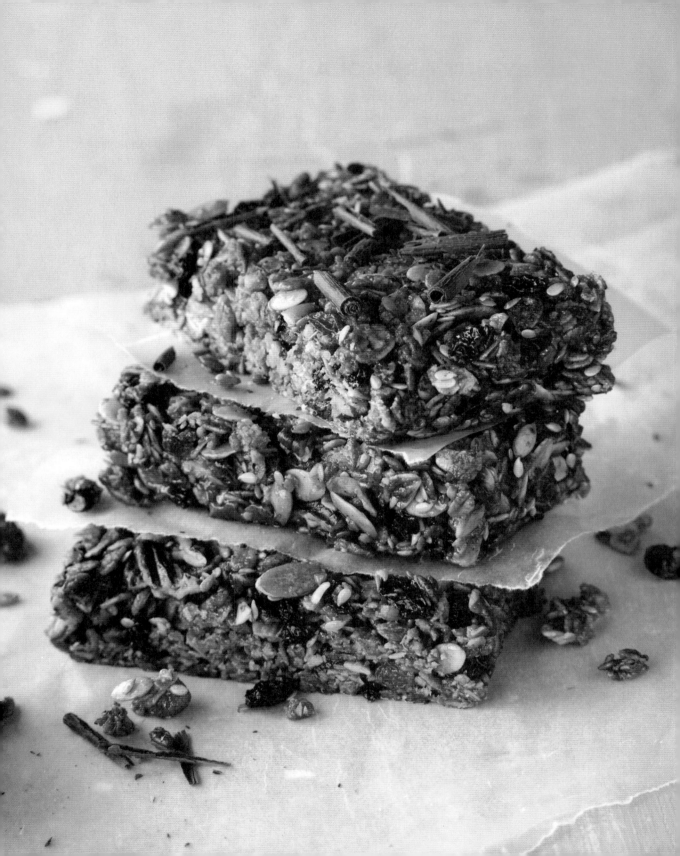

HONEY-NUT GRANOLA

GLUTEN-FREE

SERVES 8 • PREP TIME: 10 MINUTES • COOK TIME: 1½ HOURS

This recipe is just a guideline for the personalized recipe you will create to suit your palate. If you love almonds, then use them instead of hazelnuts; or add raisins or dried cherries instead of cranberries. Keep the oat-coconut base, though, because it provides a balanced flavor and pleasing texture that is the foundation of good granola.

---

6 cups large-flake gluten-free oats

2 cups shredded unsweetened coconut

1 cup raw sunflower seeds

½ cup raw pumpkin seeds

½ cup hazelnuts

¾ cup raw honey

½ cup melted coconut oil

1 teaspoon ground cinnamon

½ teaspoon ground nutmeg

1 cup dried cranberries

1. Preheat the oven to 250°F.

2. Line two baking sheets with parchment paper. Set aside.

3. In a large bowl, toss together the oats, coconut, sunflower seeds, pumpkin seeds, and hazelnuts until mixed.

4. In a small bowl, whisk the honey, coconut oil, cinnamon, and nutmeg until blended.

5. Pour the honey mixture into the oat mixture and mix using your hands until very well coated.

6. Transfer the granola mixture to the baking sheets and spread it out evenly.

7. Bake the granola, stirring frequently, until the mixture is golden brown and crunchy, about 1½ hours.

8. Transfer the granola to a large bowl and stir in the cranberries.

9. Let the granola cool, tossing it frequently to break up the large pieces.

10. Store the granola in airtight containers in the refrigerator or freezer for up to 1 month.

TIP Cranberries are most often thought of as an effective treatment for urinary tract infections, but they also can boost the immune system and reduce inflammation in the body. Cranberries are packed with dietary fiber, protein, and an impressive array of vitamins, including vitamins A, B_6, B_{12}, C, E, and K.

PEAR MUESLI

VEGAN GLUTEN-FREE

SERVES 4 • PREP TIME: 10 MINUTES PLUS CHILLING TIME • COOK TIME: 0 MINUTES

This muesli is considered to be a "fresh" version because it consists of an assortment of wholesome ingredients that are soaked overnight to soften. This comforting dish originated in Switzerland as a healthful option for patients who needed added nutrition for recovery. If you are traveling in Switzerland or Germany, you might find muesli served in the early evening as well as at breakfast.

---

2 ripe pears, cored and grated

2 cups large-flake gluten-free oats

½ cup shredded unsweetened coconut

2 cups canned coconut milk

2 tablespoons maple syrup

1 tablespoon chia seeds

1 tablespoon freshly squeezed lemon juice

½ teaspoon ground cinnamon

1. In a large sealable container, stir together the pear, oats, coconut, coconut milk, maple syrup, chia seeds, juice, and cinnamon until very well mixed.

2. Seal the container and put it in the refrigerator overnight.

3. In the morning, stir and serve.

COCONUT CHIA PORRIDGE

GLUTEN-FREE

SERVES 4 • PREP TIME: 10 MINUTES PLUS GELLING TIME • COOK TIME: 0 MINUTES

There are many hot and cold cereals that make wonderful breakfast choices, and this one with pearly chia seeds is made the night before. You can enjoy a nutritious energy-packed meal with no preparation and head out the door to face the day. Adjust the sweetness to suit your own taste and try maple syrup instead of honey if that sweetener is your favorite.

1 cup canned coconut milk

1 cup plain Greek yogurt

¼ cup chia seeds

¼ cup honey

¼ cup shredded unsweetened coconut

1 tablespoon vanilla extract

1 cup raspberries

1 cup blueberries

1. In a medium bowl, stir together the coconut milk, yogurt, chia seeds, honey, coconut, and vanilla.

2. Cover the bowl and put it in the refrigerator overnight.

3. Serve the porridge cold or warm, topped with raspberries and blueberries.

TIP Chia seeds are gathered by hand and usually put into their packaging with no additives or preservatives, just seeds. However, you should buy organic chia seeds whenever possible, since the nonorganic seeds could contain traces of chemical pesticides.

COCONUT-LEMON MUFFINS

GLUTEN-FREE

MAKES 18 MUFFINS • PREP TIME: 10 MINUTES PLUS COOLING TIME • COOK TIME: 30 MINUTES

Lemon and poppy seed is a traditional combination, but these tender muffins have the added bonus of coconut and tangy lemon yogurt. Sweet fresh berries would make a lovely addition to the citrus tartness, so add a cup of blueberries or raspberries for a pretty variation.

2 cups almond flour

1 cup shredded unsweetened coconut

¼ cup poppy seeds

1½ teaspoons baking powder

½ teaspoon baking soda

⅛ teaspoon sea salt

1 cup sugar

3 eggs

¼ cup melted coconut oil

½ cup lemon yogurt

1 tablespoon finely grated lemon zest

1. Preheat the oven to 350°F.

2. Line 18 muffin cups with paper liners. Set aside

3. In a medium bowl, whisk together the flour, coconut, poppy seeds, baking powder, baking soda, and salt until well combined.

4. In a large bowl, with an electric hand beater set on high speed, beat together the sugar, eggs, and coconut oil for 2 minutes.

5. Add the yogurt and lemon zest to the egg mixture and beat until combined, scraping down the sides of the bowl.

6. Add the dry ingredients to the wet ingredients and stir until just combined.

7. Spoon the batter into the prepared muffin tin.

8. Bake until the muffins are light golden brown and a toothpick inserted in the center comes out clean, about 30 minutes.

9. Remove the muffin tin from the oven and let the muffins cool on a wire rack for about 1 hour.

10. Store the muffins in a sealed container in the refrigerator for up to 5 days or wrap each muffin individually and store in the freezer for 2 weeks.

TIP Always scrub commercially produced lemons with a soft-bristle brush and warm water before grating the skin. Otherwise your lemon zest may contain pesticides or the wax coating that is applied to lemons to protect them during transport.

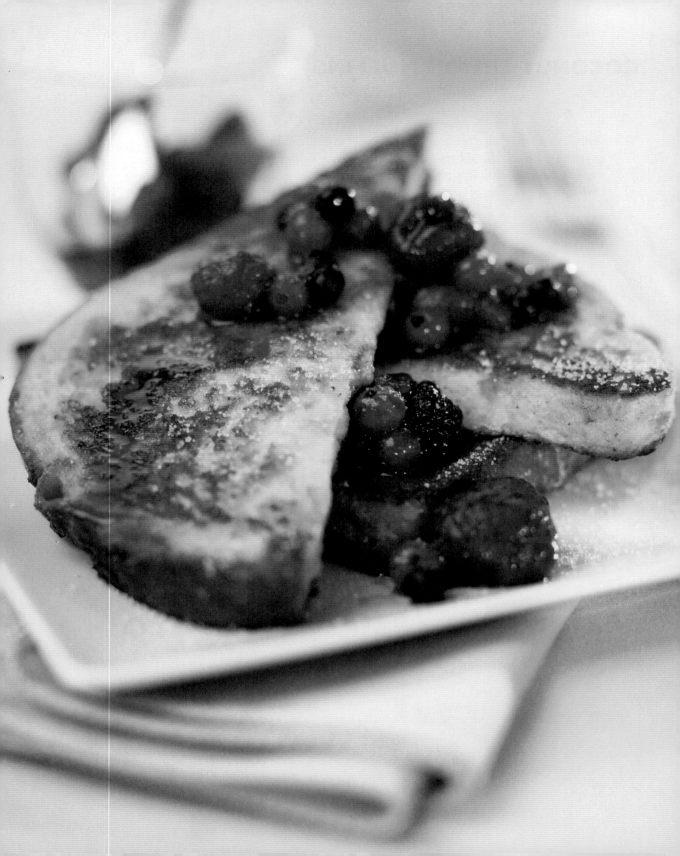

COCONUT FRENCH TOAST

SERVES 4 • PREP TIME: 15 MINUTES • COOK TIME: 25 MINUTES

Golden egg-soaked bread generously crusted with sweet coconut is the perfect choice for even the pickiest of eaters. The hint of orange in the egg mixture adds enough sweetness, so you can skip any other topping and enjoy this dish plain. If you are pressed for time, this recipe can be made ahead and reheated in a low-heat oven for about 10 minutes. Top with fresh ripe berries if they are in season for a spectacular taste and presentation.

4 large eggs

¾ cup canned coconut milk

¼ cup orange juice

1 teaspoon coconut extract

¼ teaspoon sea salt

1½ cups shredded unsweetened coconut

Coconut oil, for greasing the skillet

8 (½-inch-thick) slices French bread,

1. Preheat the oven to 225°F.

2. In a large bowl, whisk together the eggs, coconut milk, orange juice, coconut extract, and salt.

3. Spread the coconut on a large plate and set next to the egg mixture.

4. Set a skillet over medium heat and grease it lightly with coconut oil.

5. Dip the bread slices into the egg mixture, two at a time, and then dredge the soaked bread in the coconut so that both sides are well covered.

6. Fry the French toast in the skillet until golden brown on both sides, about 3 minutes per side.

7. Place the cooked French toast on a plate in the oven to keep warm while you cook the rest.

8. Repeat with all the bread slices, adding more coconut to the plate if needed.

9. Serve 2 pieces per person.

SWEET POTATO-COCONUT PANCAKES

PALEO-FRIENDLY GLUTEN-FREE

SERVES 3 • PREP TIME: 10 MINUTES • COOK TIME: 18 MINUTES

Pancakes seem like a weekend dish to be enjoyed at a leisurely breakfast or brunch with loved ones. You will feel extra special sitting down to these golden, warmly spiced beauties, especially if you have real maple syrup to drizzle over a big stack. You can add a sprinkling of chopped pecans or dollop of whipped cream if you are feeling truly decadent.

1½ cups almond flour

2 teaspoons baking powder

1 teaspoon cinnamon

½ teaspoon ginger

½ teaspoon sea salt

¼ teaspoon ground nutmeg

1 cup canned coconut milk

½ cup mashed sweet potato

2 tablespoons honey

2 tablespoons melted coconut oil

1 egg

Nonstick spray for greasing the skillet

Butter (optional)

Maple syrup (optional)

1. In a large bowl, stir together the almond flour, baking powder, cinnamon, ginger, salt, and nutmeg until mixed.

2. In a medium bowl, whisk the coconut milk, sweet potato, honey, coconut oil, and egg until well blended with no lumps.

3. Stir the wet ingredients into the dry ingredients until just combined.

4. Set a large skillet over medium heat and coat it with cooking spray.

5. When the skillet is hot, spoon the pancake batter into it, ¼ cup per pancake.

6. Cook the pancakes until golden brown, about 3 minutes per side.

7. Serve 2 pancakes per person with butter and syrup (if using).

GOLDEN COCONUT WAFFLES

SERVES 6 • PREP TIME: 10 MINUTES • COOK TIME: 20 MINUTES

The addition of buttermilk creates a tender waffle that cooks up golden and crispy every time. You can still enjoy these delicious waffles even if you do not own a waffle maker. Simply whip up the recipe and use a greased skillet to make golden coconut pancakes instead. If the batter is too thin for perfect pancakes, add a little more flour until you have the right consistency.

1 cup shredded unsweetened coconut

1 cup all-purpose flour

½ cup almond flour

½ cup arrowroot powder

½ cup sugar

1 teaspoon baking powder

½ teaspoon baking soda

½ teaspoon sea salt

2 large eggs

1 cup canned coconut milk, at room temperature

1 cup buttermilk, at room temperature

½ cup coconut oil, melted

Nonstick cooking oil spray

Butter (optional)

Maple syrup (optional)

Fresh fruit (optional)

1. In a large bowl, stir together the coconut, all-purpose flour, almond flour, arrowroot powder, sugar, baking powder, baking soda, and salt.

2. In a medium bowl, whisk together the eggs, coconut milk, buttermilk, and coconut oil until well blended.

3. Stir the wet ingredients into the dry ingredients until just combined.

4. Heat a waffle iron until very hot. Spray the iron lightly with nonstick spray.

5. Working in batches, cook the waffles until golden brown.

6. Serve 2 waffles per person, topped with butter, syrup, or fresh fruit (if using).

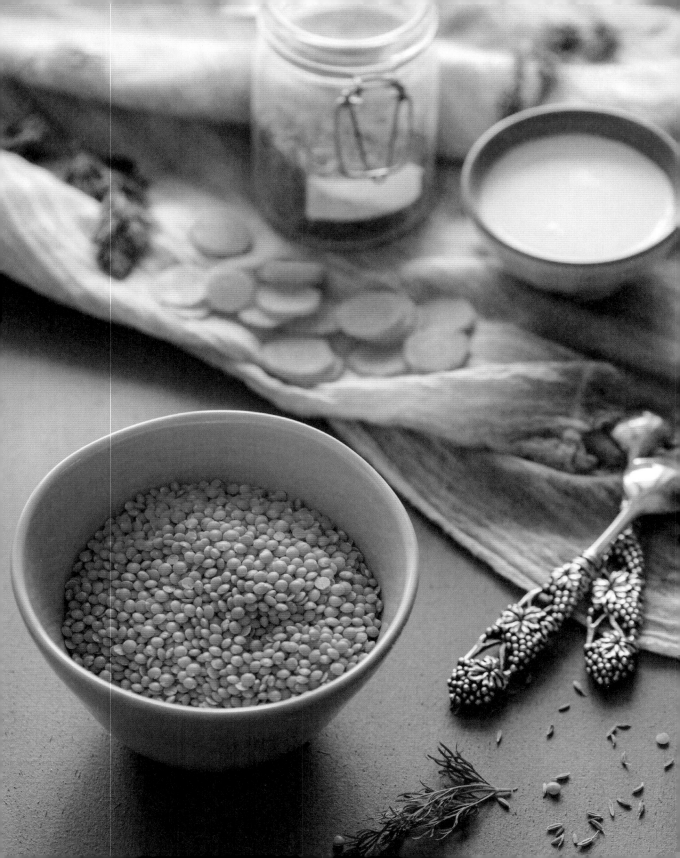

Chapter Eight

SOUPS & SALADS

SPICY COCONUT QUINOA BOWL

GLUTEN-FREE

SERVES 4 • PREP TIME: 20 MINUTES • COOK TIME: 10 MINUTES

Hot jalapeño pepper adds a fair amount of heat to this flavorful Asian-themed lunch bowl, because it contains a compound called capsaicin. The coconut milk and heaps of vegetables in the dish help cut the heat a little, so do not be afraid that it will be scorching. If you enjoy hot food, you can turn the heat up by substituting a fierier pepper such as habanero or Scotch bonnet.

---

3 garlic cloves

2 shallots, peeled

2 teaspoons grated fresh ginger

1 jalapeño pepper, seeded and minced

Juice and zest of 1 lime

1 tablespoon coconut oil

2 cups canned coconut milk

1 tablespoon coconut aminos

1 tablespoon honey

3 cups cooked quinoa

1 cup shredded carrot

1 cup julienned snow peas

1 red bell pepper, julienned

1 cup bean sprouts

Chopped fresh cilantro, for garnish

1. Put the garlic, shallots, ginger, jalapeño pepper, lime juice and zest, and coconut oil in a blender and blend until a smooth paste.

2. Add the coconut milk, coconut aminos, and honey to the blender and blend until combined, for one minute.

3. Pour the sauce mixture into a saucepan and set it over medium heat.

4. Bring the mixture to a boil, then reduce the heat to low and simmer for 10 minutes.

5. Remove the sauce from the heat and set aside.

6. Put the quinoa, carrot, snow peas, red pepper, and sprouts in a large bowl and toss to mix.

7. Add the sauce and stir to combine.

8. Serve the quinoa bowl topped with cilantro.

TIP If you are looking to increase the amount of protein in your diet, quinoa should be at the top of your list of foods to include. Quinoa is considered a complete protein because it contains all nine essential amino acids. Quinoa is also a marvelous source of calcium, iron, and amino acids such as lysine.

CHICKEN-CHILI SOUP

PALEO-FRIENDLY GLUTEN-FREE

SERVES 6 • PREP TIME: 15 MINUTES • COOK TIME: 20 MINUTES

Frigid winter days will somehow feel less cold when you tuck into this chili-infused soup. Chunks of tender chicken, sweet carrot, and shreds of cabbage nestle in spicy lime-spiked broth, creating an adventure for your palate that will warm you right down to your toes. You can change up the vegetables in this recipe easily and add a can of diced tomato if you need more portions for company or to freeze for a future meal.

---

1 tablespoon coconut oil

1 sweet onion, peeled and chopped

1 tablespoon minced garlic

2 teaspoons grated fresh ginger

4 cups cooked diced chicken

2 cups diced carrot

2 cups shredded cabbage

6 cups chicken broth

2 cups canned coconut milk

½ cup shredded unsweetened coconut

1½ tablespoons red chili paste or as desired

Zest and juice of 1 lime

2 cups shredded kale

1. Set a large stockpot over medium-high heat and add the coconut oil.

2. Sauté the onion, garlic, and ginger until softened, about 3 minutes.

3. Add the chicken, carrot, cabbage, broth, coconut milk, coconut, chili paste, and lime juice and zest to the stock pot.

4. Bring the soup to a boil and then reduce the heat to low and simmer until the carrots are tender, for 10 minutes.

5. Stir in the kale and serve.

CARROT-COCONUT SOUP

VEGAN GLUTEN-FREE

SERVES 6 • PREP TIME: 15 MINUTES • COOK TIME: 40 MINUTES

Carrots are the main ingredient in this sunny soup, so it is important to get the best produce possible. Look for carrots that are brightly colored with the greens attached if possible. Just make sure you remove the greens before storing your carrots, or the cores will dry out. Avoid carrots with cracks, and choose vegetables with wider diameters, because those carrots are usually sweeter.

---

1 tablespoon coconut oil

1 medium sweet onion, peeled and chopped

1 teaspoon minced garlic

1 teaspoon grated fresh ginger

6 carrots, peeled and chopped

1 cup peeled and diced potatoes

5 cups chicken stock

1 cup canned coconut milk

1 teaspoon ground cumin

Sea salt

Freshly ground black pepper

1. In a large pot, heat the coconut oil over medium heat.
2. Add the onion, garlic, and ginger and sauté until translucent, about 4 minutes.
3. Add the carrots, potatoes, stock, coconut milk, and cumin.
4. Bring the soup to a boil, then reduce the heat to low and simmer the soup until the vegetables are soft, about 30 minutes.
5. Purée the soup in batches in a food processor until smooth.
6. Return the puréed soup to the pot and season with salt and pepper.
7. Serve.

BUTTERNUT SQUASH-COCONUT BOWL

VEGAN

SERVES 4 • PREP TIME: 10 MINUTES • COOK TIME: 15 MINUTES

This is a magnificent dish that has texture, color, and a multitude of complementary flavors all in one bowl. Barley adds a nutty taste and pasta-like consistency along with a healthful dose of fiber to help promote food digestion and stable blood sugar. Barley can sometimes have tiny rocks in the package so take the time to rinse this grain and pick through it before using it in this bowl.

---

1 pound butternut squash, peeled, seeded, and cut into ½-inch chunks

2 cups cooked barley

1 cup cooked red lentils

1 scallion, chopped

½ cup shredded unsweetened coconut

½ cup pumpkin seeds

3 tablespoons chopped fresh cilantro

¼ cup melted coconut oil

2 tablespoons balsamic vinegar

Sea salt

Freshly ground black pepper

1. Put the squash in a saucepan filled with water and bring to a boil over medium-high heat.

2. Reduce the heat to low and simmer the squash until it is tender, about 15 minutes.

3. Drain the squash and transfer it to a large bowl.

4. Add the barley, lentils, scallion, coconut, pumpkin seeds, and cilantro to the squash and stir to combine.

5. Whisk the coconut oil and balsamic vinegar together and add the dressing to the bowl.

6. Stir to combine and season with salt and pepper.

7. Serve slightly warm or chilled.

RED LENTIL–COCONUT SOUP

VEGAN GLUTEN-FREE

SERVES 6 • PREP TIME: 15 MINUTES • COOK TIME: 1 HOUR

Lentil soup seems like a humble offering, which is accurate because at one time only peasants would eat this unassuming legume. Lentils make a superb soup ingredient because they soak up seasonings like a sponge and can be either cooked to a thick consistency or just cooked enough to remain whole but tender. If you want to save a little time, you can substitute sodium-free canned lentils for the dried lentils in this recipe. Add them with all the other ingredients, cut the chicken stock by 4 cups and reduce the cooking time by about 20 minutes.

---

2 tablespoons coconut oil, divided

2 large potatoes, peeled and diced small

1 tablespoon minced garlic

1 small onion, peeled and chopped

2 celery stalks, chopped with the greens

3 cups red lentils, washed, picked over, and drained

7 cups vegetable broth

1 cup canned coconut milk

Sea salt

Freshly ground black pepper

2 tablespoons coarsely chopped fresh cilantro

1. Set a large pot on medium-high heat and add half the coconut oil.

2. Sauté the potatoes until they are tender and lightly golden, about 6 minutes.

3. Remove the potatoes with a slotted spoon to a paper towel–covered plate and set aside.

4. Place the pot back on the heat and add the remaining coconut oil.

5. Sauté the garlic, onion, and celery until the vegetables are translucent, about 4 minutes.

6. Add the lentils and the broth.

7. Bring the soup to a boil and then reduce the heat to low and simmer the soup until the lentils are soft and the soup is thick, about 45 minutes.

8. Remove the pot from the heat and purée the soup with an immersion blender or in a food processor until smooth.

9. Transfer the soup back to the pot.

10. Whisk in the coconut milk and season with salt and pepper.

11. Serve topped with the fried potatoes and cilantro.

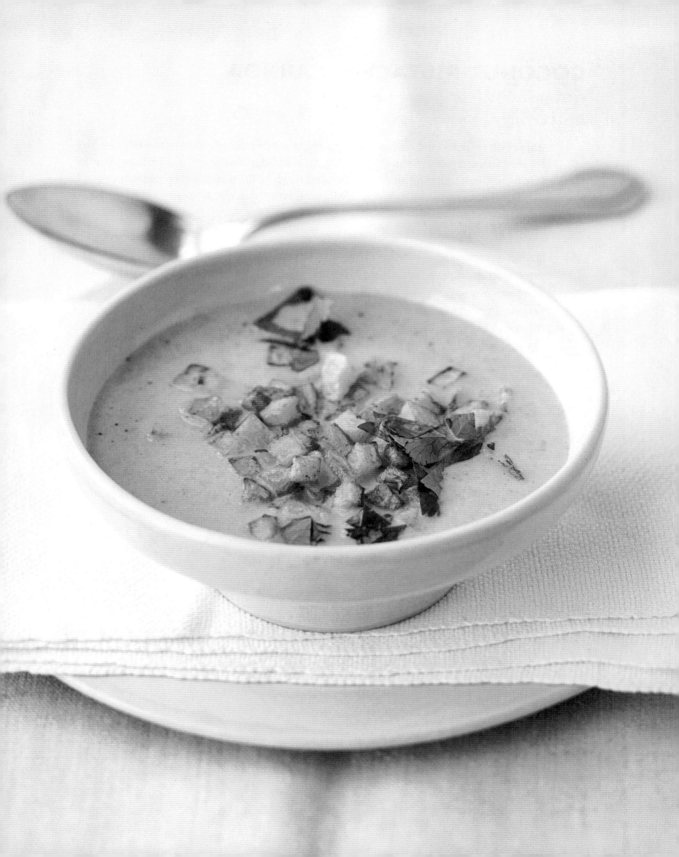

COCONUT-PISTACHIO QUINOA

VEGAN GLUTEN-FREE

SERVES 4 • PREP TIME: 10 MINUTES • COOK TIME: 30 MINUTES

Simple can be better when you do not want to make a lot of effort in the kitchen but still want a satisfying meal. Quinoa cooks up quickly and combines brilliantly with most ingredients, including pistachios and fresh herbs. Unsalted pistachios are best, but if your nuts are salted, you might want to skip the seasoning step at the end of the recipe.

---

1 tablespoon coconut oil

1 small sweet onion, peeled and minced

2 teaspoons minced garlic

2 teaspoons grated fresh ginger

2 (15-ounce) cans coconut milk

1 cup quinoa, rinsed and drained

2 scallions, chopped

¼ cup shredded unsweetened coconut

¼ cup chopped pistachios

Sea salt

2 tablespoons chopped fresh cilantro

1. Set a large saucepan over medium-high heat and melt the coconut oil.

2. Sauté the onion, garlic, and ginger until the vegetables are soft, about 4 minutes.

3. Add the coconut milk and quinoa. Bring the mixture to a boil and reduce the heat to low.

4. Simmer the quinoa, covered, stirring occasionally, until the quinoa is tender, about 20 minutes.

5. Stir in the scallions, coconut, and pistachios.

6. Season with salt and serve topped with cilantro.

TIP Ginger is a centuries-old remedy for nausea and other digestive issues because it is an anti-inflammatory. Herbal medicine recommends the use of ginger for ailments such as heartburn, migraines, and joint inflammation. Modern studies have concluded that ginger is also effective for reducing the risk of some cancers, including ovarian and colon cancer.

CURRIED CABBAGE SLAW

GLUTEN-FREE

SERVES 6 • PREP TIME: 25 MINUTES PLUS CHILLING TIME • COOK TIME: 0 MINUTES

This dish is not your usual picnic-style coleslaw; it is studded with dried fruit, and the dressing is warmly spiced with lemony coriander and a touch of curry. Similar to other coleslaw recipes, this one gets better as it sits because the cabbage and kale absorb the dressing and the flavor mellows. If you have leftover salad, it makes a delectable sandwich topping on shaved beef or shredded pork.

½ head napa cabbage, shredded

½ head red cabbage, shredded

2 cups shredded kale

2 large carrots, peeled and shredded

½ red onion, thinly sliced

1 cup shredded unsweetened coconut

½ cup dried cranberries

½ cup canned coconut milk

¼ cup sour cream

2 tablespoons fresh lemon juice

1 tablespoon granulated sugar

1 teaspoon ground cumin

½ teaspoon good-quality curry powder

¼ teaspoon coriander

Sea salt

1. In a large bowl, toss together the cabbages, kale, carrots, red onion, coconut, and cranberries until well mixed.

2. In a small bowl, whisk the coconut milk, sour cream, lemon juice, sugar, cumin, curry, and coriander until blended.

3. Add the dressing to the cabbage mixture and toss to mix.

4. Season with salt.

5. Let the cabbage slaw sit covered in the refrigerator for 2 hours to allow the flavors to mellow.

6. Serve.

7. Store leftovers for up to 3 days in the refrigerator.

COCONUT–WHEAT BERRY SALAD

VEGAN

SERVES 6 • PREP TIME: 20 MINUTES • COOK TIME: 1 HOUR

Wheat berries are the entire wheat kernel, endosperm, bran, and germ. When you use whole-wheat flour, you are using the processed form of wheat berries. Wheat berries have a lovely nutty taste and an interesting, slightly chewy texture when cooked, so they are absolutely delicious in salads and side dishes as an alternative to other grains and legumes. This tasty ingredient is high in protein, fiber, and B vitamins.

2 cups wheat berries

7 cups water

2 cups shredded unsweetened coconut

1 cup diced extra-firm tofu

1 tomato, diced

1 cup pomegranate seeds

½ red onion, diced

¼ cup chopped fresh cilantro

¼ cup sliced almonds

Juice of 3 limes

Sea salt

Freshly ground black pepper

1. Place a large saucepan filled with 7 cups of water over medium-high heat. Add the wheat berries and bring to a boil.

2. Reduce the heat to low and simmer, covered, for 1 hour, until the wheat berries are soft and chewy.

3. When the wheat berries are cool, add the coconut, tofu, tomato, pomegranate seeds, red onion, cilantro, sliced almonds, and lime juice to the bowl. Toss to mix.

4. Season with salt and pepper.

5. Serve.

TIP   You can cook the wheat berries ahead of time and store them in the refrigerator for up to 2 days in a sealed container until you put together the salad. You can even freeze this grain for up to 1 month.

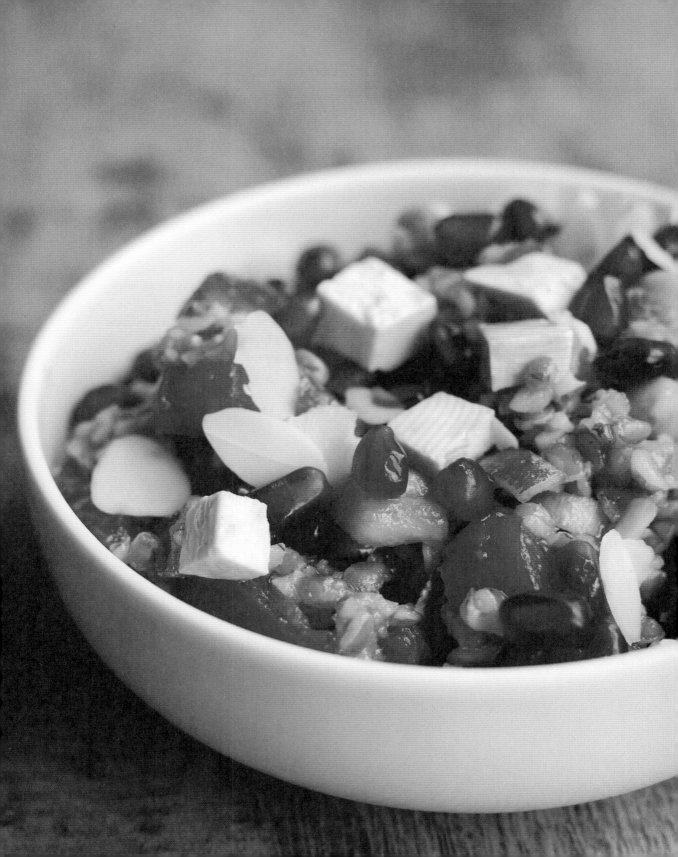

FRUIT SALAD WITH TROPICAL COCONUT DRESSING

PALEO-FRIENDLY **VEGAN** GLUTEN-FREE

SERVES 4 • PREP TIME: 20 MINUTES • COOK TIME: 0 MINUTES

When you see the gorgeous golden dressing you will be using for your salad, the day will seem a little brighter, and you will not be able to wait for lunch. If ripe mango is not available for your recipe, you can use frozen mango. Papaya can be substituted if you want a deeper-hued vinaigrette.

For the dressing
¾ cup canned coconut milk
1 mango, peeled, pitted, and chopped
1 tablespoon coconut oil
¼ cup freshly squeezed lime juice
Pinch sea salt

For the salad
4 cups chopped kale, washed and dried
2 cups diced pineapple
1 large papaya, peeled, seeded, and diced
2 kiwifruits, peeled and diced
1 cup shredded unsweetened coconut

To make the dressing

1. Put the coconut milk, mango, coconut oil, and lime juice in a blender and blend until smooth.

2. Season with salt and set aside.

To make the salad

1. In a large bowl, toss the kale with the dressing and arrange the leaves on 4 plates.

2. In a medium bowl, toss together the pineapple, papaya, and kiwifruits and top the salad evenly with the fruit.

3. Sprinkle the salad with the shredded coconut and serve.

TIP Kiwifruit adds a lovely pale green accent to salads as well as a hefty nutritional punch. Kiwifruit is a wonderful source of vitamins A, C, and E, as well as fiber, potassium, and antioxidants. This fruit can promote eye health, boost immunity, and reduce the risk of asthma.

GREEN MANGO SALAD WITH CURRY COCONUT DRESSING

VEGAN GLUTEN-FREE

SERVES 4 • PREP TIME: 30 MINUTES • COOK TIME: 0 MINUTES

The combination of green and ripe mangoes is exotic, and the different textures are a pleasure. This meal-size salad is magnificent looking, with fresh, vibrant colors and a citrus-spiked peanut dressing. You can add a grilled chicken breast or piece of white-fleshed fish for a more substantial meal.

For the dressing

1 cup canned coconut milk

¼ cup peanut butter

¼ cup freshly squeezed lime juice

1 teaspoon grated fresh ginger

1 tablespoon good-quality curry powder

¼ teaspoon sea salt

For the salad

3 cups shredded kale

1 green mango, peeled, pitted, and julienned

1 ripe mango, peeled, pitted, and julienned

1 red bell pepper, julienned

1 carrot, shredded

½ jicama, peeled and julienned

3 scallions, chopped

½ cup shredded unsweetened coconut

¼ cup chopped fresh cilantro, for garnish

To make the dressing

1. In a small bowl, whisk together the coconut milk, peanut butter, lime juice, ginger, curry powder, and salt.

2. Set aside.

To make the salad

1. In a large bowl, toss the kale, mangoes, red pepper, carrot, jicama, scallions, and coconut until well mixed.

2. Add the dressing and toss to coat.

3. Serve topped with cilantro.

TIP The fruit and vegetables in this dish need to be julienned in order to get the right texture, and all that knife work can take a lot of time. A mandoline can save you some serious prep time if you like recipes with lots of cut produce. This kitchen tool has perpendicular and parallel blades that can cut your produce into slices, julienned strips, crosshatched pieces, and batons.

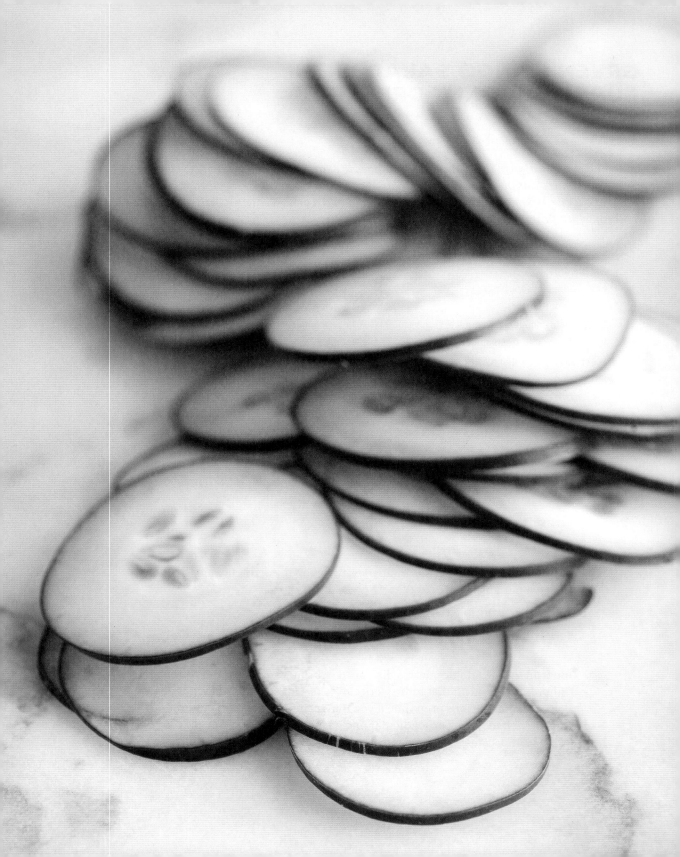

Chapter Nine

SNACKS & APPETIZERS

STRAWBERRY-VANILLA SPREAD

PALEO-FRIENDLY VEGAN GLUTEN-FREE

MAKES 3 CUPS • PREP TIME: 25 MINUTES • COOK TIME: 0 MINUTES

Looking for a delicious spread or tasty dip? Look no further than this pastel-pink vanilla-scented butter. Fresh coconut is usually available in the produce section of the grocery store, and picking a perfect one is quite easy. A coconut should be uniformly brown and feel heavier than it looks from the size. When you shake the coconut, you should hear sloshing from the coconut milk inside. If you do not hear the water, this means there might be a crack that allowed the water to drain out.

2 cups shredded fresh coconut

1½ cups fresh strawberries

2 tablespoons maple syrup

½ tablespoon freshly squeezed lemon juice

½ tablespoon pure vanilla extract

½ tablespoon coconut oil

1. Put the coconut in a food processor and purée until it has a butter-like consistency, about 15 minutes.

2. Add the strawberries, maple syrup, lemon juice, vanilla, and coconut oil to the coconut butter and process until very smooth, scraping down the sides at least twice.

3. Press the butter through a very fine sieve using the back of a spoon to remove the strawberry seeds.

4. Store the butter in the refrigerator for up to 2 weeks.

5. Let it soften at room temperature before using it as a spread.

CREAMY VANILLA-COCONUT YOGURT

PALEO-FRIENDLY GLUTEN-FREE

MAKES 3 CUPS • PREP TIME: 25 MINUTES PLUS FERMENTING TIME • COOK TIME: 0 MINUTES

Making yogurt is not difficult if you have probiotic powder to create the delicious tangy taste. You can find this powder in capsules in the supplements section of the supermarket. Yogurt can replenish the friendly bacteria in your digestive tract, which promotes better digestion and boosts the immune system. Try to eat probiotic yogurt every day to keep adequate amounts of bacteria in your body.

---

2 cups chopped fresh coconut

1 cup coconut water

2 tablespoons honey

2 teaspoons pure vanilla extract

½ teaspoon probiotic powder

1. Put the coconut and coconut water in a food processor and process until very smooth and creamy, about 10 minutes.

2. Add the honey and vanilla and process until well blended, scraping down the sides.

3. Add the probiotic powder and process until it is blended into the mixture.

4. Transfer the vanilla yogurt to a container with a lid.

5. Store the yogurt in the refrigerator for at least 18 hours until it tastes like yogurt.

6. Keep in the refrigerator for up to 1 week.

CLASSIC AMBROSIA

GLUTEN-FREE

SERVES 4 • PREP TIME: 15 MINUTES PLUS CHILLING TIME • COOK TIME: 0 MINUTES

You will not see the traditional version of this recipe gracing tables of people counting calories or trying to avoid sweets. Ambrosia is rich and decadent and has a light, airy texture. This is truly a food of the gods as the name implies. To save time, you can use canned pineapple and mandarin oranges, or instead of fresh fruit, use a big can of fruit salad packed in fruit juice.

½ cup heavy (whipping) cream

½ cup sour cream

3 cups mini-marshmallows

1 cup chopped fresh pineapple

3 Clementine tangerines, peeled and segmented, wedges cut in half

1½ cups shredded fresh coconut

1 cup chopped pecans

1. In a large bowl using an electric hand beater on medium speed, whip the cream until it forms stiff peaks.

2. Stir in the sour cream, marshmallows, pineapple, tangerines, coconut, and pecans until well mixed.

3. Put the bowl in the refrigerator for 3 hours to set, and serve.

TIP Pineapple is one of those foods that tastes like it smells—sweet and lush. You should be able to hold a pineapple up to your nose in the grocery store and smell that fragrance. If you cannot, put the pineapple back, because it is not ripe enough. Since pineapple does not continue to ripen after it is picked, it is important to get a ripe one right from the store.

CREAMY COCONUT FRUIT DIP

GLUTEN-FREE

MAKES 5 SERVINGS • PREP TIME: 10 MINUTES • COOK TIME: 0 MINUTES

Seeing a dip with a platter of cut-up vegetables is quite common, but fruit plates often exclude this enhancement. You might never serve fruit alone again after trying this fluffy, tangy dip. The hint of warm cinnamon elevates the taste to something sublime. The cream cheese should be very soft when beating it with the other ingredients, or your dip will end up lumpy.

½ cup heavy (whipping) cream

1 tablespoon granulated sugar

4 ounces canned coconut cream

2 ounces cream cheese, softened

1 teaspoon coconut oil

¼ teaspoon ground cinnamon

1. In a medium bowl using an electric hand beater on medium speed, whip the cream and sugar until stiff peaks form. Set aside.

2. In another medium bowl, use the hand beater to whip the coconut cream, cream cheese, coconut oil, and cinnamon until very smooth.

3. Fold the whipped cream into the coconut cream mixture until well combined.

4. Store covered in the refrigerator for up to 2 days and serve with cut-up fruit.

CUCUMBER-COCONUT DIP

PALEO-FRIENDLY VEGAN GLUTEN-FREE

MAKES 4 CUPS • PREP TIME: 25 MINUTES • COOK TIME: 0 MINUTES

Cool, creamy, herb-infused dips can be used for vegetables, breads, crackers, and as a tasty sandwich spread. This dip features fresh cilantro and a splash of lemon juice to perk up your taste buds. Cilantro contains a natural chemical compound called aldehyde that some people are genetically predisposed to find unpleasant. But if you like this herb you're in luck; it is high in magnesium and iron, which can fight anemia and combat arthritis.

---

4 cups fresh coconut

Juice from ½ lemon

1 teaspoon minced garlic

½ English cucumber, diced

½ tablespoon finely chopped fresh cilantro

1 teaspoon ground coriander

½ teaspoon cumin

Sea salt

Freshly ground black pepper

1 tablespoon chopped mint, for garnish

½ teaspoon olive oil, for garnish

1. Process the coconut, lemon juice, and garlic in a food processor until very smooth, scraping down the sides, about 10 minutes.

2. Transfer the coconut mixture to a bowl and stir in the cucumber, cilantro, coriander, and cumin.

3. Season with salt and pepper.

4. Top with mint and a drizzle of olive oil.

5. Serve with vegetables or crackers.

TIP   Cilantro is one of the herbs that can get limp and moldy very quickly in your refrigerator, and it is sold in huge bunches. Rather than constantly throw away your unused cilantro, try freezing it to preserve the taste and freshness. Place sprigs of cilantro on a baking sheet in the freezer and when it is completely frozen, transfer the sprigs to sealable freezer bags. Freeze this herb for up to 3 months.

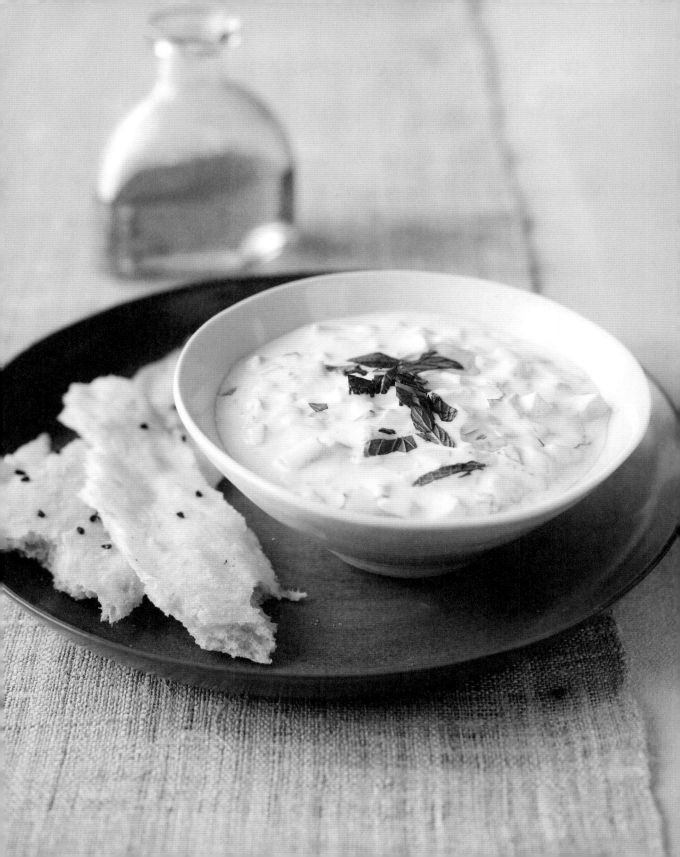

SPICE-ROASTED CHICKPEAS

VEGAN GLUTEN-FREE

MAKES 4 CUPS • PREP TIME: 10 MINUTES • COOK TIME: 30 MINUTES

Sometimes an occasion calls out for a crunchy, spicy snack, and it is unhealthy to reach for chips and other processed choices all the time. Roasted chickpeas are crispy, nutty tasting, and simple to create quickly in your own oven. Try different spice combinations, such as herbs, chili, and sea salt, until you find a favorite flavor.

2 (15-ounce) cans sodium-free chickpeas, drained, rinsed, and thoroughly dried

¼ cup coconut oil, melted

1 teaspoon sea salt

1 teaspoon ground cumin

½ teaspoon ground coriander

½ teaspoon ground ginger

¼ teaspoon smoked paprika

Pinch cayenne pepper

1. Preheat the oven to 425°F.

2. Line a baking sheet with parchment paper and set aside.

3. In a large bowl, toss the chickpeas in the coconut oil until well coated

4. Add the sea salt, cumin, coriander, ginger, smoked paprika, and cayenne pepper to the bowl. Toss well to combine.

5. Spread the chickpeas in a single layer on the baking sheet and put the sheet in the oven.

6. Roast the chickpeas, stirring once, until they are crunchy and golden, about 30 minutes.

7. Let them cool and store in a sealed container in the refrigerator for up to 1 week.

TIP In order to ensure a delectable, crunchy snack, you must completely dry the chickpeas before tossing them with the other ingredients. The oil will not evenly coat the chickpeas if there is a smidge of moisture on them.

GARLICKY COCONUT KALE CHIPS

PALEO-FRIENDLY VEGAN GLUTEN-FREE

SERVES 4 • PREP TIME: 10 MINUTES • COOK TIME: 25 MINUTES

Kale chips are a phenomenon in many culinary circles because they are crunchy, can be seasoned with almost any type of spice, herb, or flavoring, and are healthy. The trick to perfect kale chips is to make sure the chopped kale is perfectly dry before adding the oil and to massage the oil into the kale evenly so that there are no uncoated spots.

---

4 cups kale

2 tablespoons coconut oil, melted

½ teaspoon minced garlic

¼ teaspoon sea salt

1. Preheat the oven to 300°F.

2. Line two baking sheets with parchment paper and set aside.

3. Remove the stems from the kale and tear the leaves into 2-inch pieces as uniformly as possible.

4. Wash the kale and dry it completely either with paper towels or in a salad spinner.

5. Transfer the kale to a large bowl and set aside.

6. Put the coconut oil and garlic in a small bowl and use the back of a spoon to crush the garlic into the coconut oil. Try to get this mixture as smooth as possible with no larger garlic chunks.

7. Add the oil mixture to the kale pieces.

8. Using your hands, toss the kale with the oil mixture to coat each leaf evenly.

9. Season with salt and toss well to combine.

10. Divide the kale evenly between the two prepared baking sheets and spread it out in a single layer on each sheet.

11. Bake until the kale chips are crispy and dry, 20 to 25 minutes, rotating the baking sheets at least once.

12. Remove the baking sheets from the oven and allow the chips to cool for about 5 minutes before serving them.

TIP Let the kale sit for at least 5 minutes after chopping it or tearing it up. When you "wound" the leaves, they produce antioxidants to repair the damage, which increases the benefits of this healthful green.

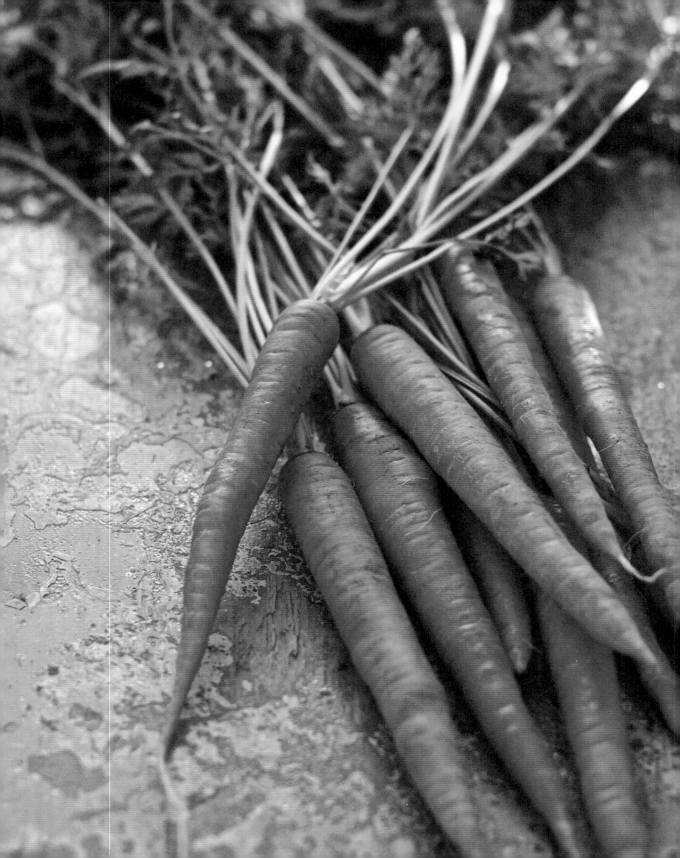

Chapter Ten

VEGAN & VEGETARIAN ENTRÉES

CORN & COCONUT CHOWDER

PALEO-FRIENDLY VEGAN GLUTEN-FREE

SERVES 4 • PREP TIME: 15 MINUTES • COOK TIME: 35 MINUTES

A chowder is a creamy soup usually thickened with flour and named for the French word for pot—chaudiere. *This recipe does not use flour because the coconut milk thickens the broth without any further additions. Corn is a traditional ingredient in chowders because it is sweet and starchy, making a substantial meal without meat or seafood. If corn is in season, you can use fresh instead of frozen.*

2 tablespoons coconut oil	4 cups corn kernels
1 sweet onion, finely diced	2 cups vegetable broth
2 teaspoons minced garlic	2 cups canned full-fat coconut milk
3 celery stalks, diced	Sea salt
1 carrot, peeled and diced	Freshly ground black pepper
1 red chile, finely diced	¼ cup chopped fresh parsley, for garnish

1. Set a large saucepan over medium-high heat and add the coconut oil.
2. Sauté the onion and garlic until softened, for 3 minutes.
3. Add the celery, carrot, and chile and sauté for an additional 3 minutes.
4. Stir in the corn, vegetable broth, and coconut milk.
5. Bring the soup to a boil and then reduce the heat to low and simmer until the vegetables are tender, about 30 minutes.
6. Remove 2 cups of soup, including some of the vegetables, and purée in a blender until smooth.
7. Pour the puréed soup back into the pot and stir to combine.
8. Season with salt and pepper.
9. Serve the soup topped with parsley.

CREAMY VEGETABLE STEW

VEGAN GLUTEN-FREE

SERVES 4 • PREP TIME: 15 MINUTES • COOK TIME: 35 MINUTES

Stews are traditionally made with meat chunks, vegetables, and a flavorful sauce. This recipe is creamy instead, with chunks of tomato for an unusual fresh taste. This stew has many ingredients that promote glowing health, such as tomatoes, peppers, carrots, kidney beans, and butternut squash. It's also a stellar source of protein and fiber, and it is full of disease-fighting antioxidants.

---

1 tablespoon coconut oil

1 sweet onion, peeled and chopped

2 teaspoons minced garlic

1 teaspoon ground cumin

1 teaspoon ground coriander

2 cups diced butternut squash

2 carrots, peeled and chopped

½ celeriac, peeled and diced

1 cup vegetable broth

1 cup canned coconut milk

2 large tomatoes, chopped

2 red bell peppers, seeded and chopped

1 cup cooked kidney beans

1 tablespoon fresh lemon juice

Pinch of hot red pepper flakes

2 tablespoons chopped fresh parsley, for garnish

1. Set a large pot over medium-high heat and add the coconut oil.

2. Sauté the onion and garlic until softened, for 3 minutes.

3. Add the cumin and coriander and stir for 1 minute.

4. Stir in the squash, carrots, and celeriac and sauté for 5 minutes.

5. Stir in the vegetable broth, coconut milk, tomatoes, and peppers.

6. Bring the vegetable stew to a boil and then reduce the heat to low so that it simmers.

7. Simmer the stew until the vegetables are tender, stirring often, about 20 minutes.

8. Add the kidney beans, lemon juice, and red pepper flakes and simmer an additional 5 minutes.

9. Serve topped with parsley.

ROOT VEGETABLE MÉLANGE

PALEO-FRIENDLY **VEGAN** GLUTEN-FREE

SERVES 4 • PREP TIME: 20 MINUTES • COOK TIME: 45 MINUTES

Root vegetables soak up whatever flavorings they are cooked, in which makes them perfect for spicy sauces. This sauce is hot because of the ginger, but it is also quite delicate with a hint of honey. If you like heat, a sprinkling of red chili flakes will create a hotter sauce without ruining the balance of flavors. You can also try butternut squash, celeriac, and parsnips for an appealing change.

---

1 cup canned coconut milk

3 tablespoons coconut aminos

3 tablespoons honey

2 teaspoons grated fresh ginger

1 teaspoon minced garlic

1 teaspoon chopped fresh thyme

1 sweet potato, peeled and cut into ½-inch chunks

1 potato, peeled and cut into ½-inch chunks

1 orange carrot, peeled and cut into ½-inch chunks

1 yellow carrot, peeled and cut into ½-inch chunks

2 beets, peeled and cut into eighths

2 shallots, peeled

½ jicama, peeled and cut into ½-inch chunks

3 tablespoons coconut oil, melted

½ cup shredded coconut

1. Preheat the oven to 375°F.

2. In a small saucepan set over medium-high heat, whisk together the coconut milk, coconut aminos, honey, ginger, and garlic until well combined.

3. Bring the sauce to a boil, reduce the heat to low, and simmer until the sauce thickens, about 5 minutes.

4. Remove the pan from the heat and stir in the thyme. Set aside.

5. To a large bowl, add the sweet potato, potato, carrots, beets, shallots, and jicama and toss with the coconut oil until the vegetables are well coated.

6. Transfer the vegetables to a large baking dish and bake them in the oven until the vegetables are lightly golden and tender, about 40 minutes.

7. Remove from the oven and serve, drizzled with the sauce and sprinkled with the shredded coconut.

TIP Jicama is an unusual-looking vegetable that resembles a bulbous potato and has crisp, sweet flesh that will remind you of a pear. Jicama contains powerful antioxidants and anti-inflammatories that fight disease and promote a healthy immune system. This delicious vegetable is high in calcium, fiber, potassium, iron, and vitamin C, while being almost fat free.

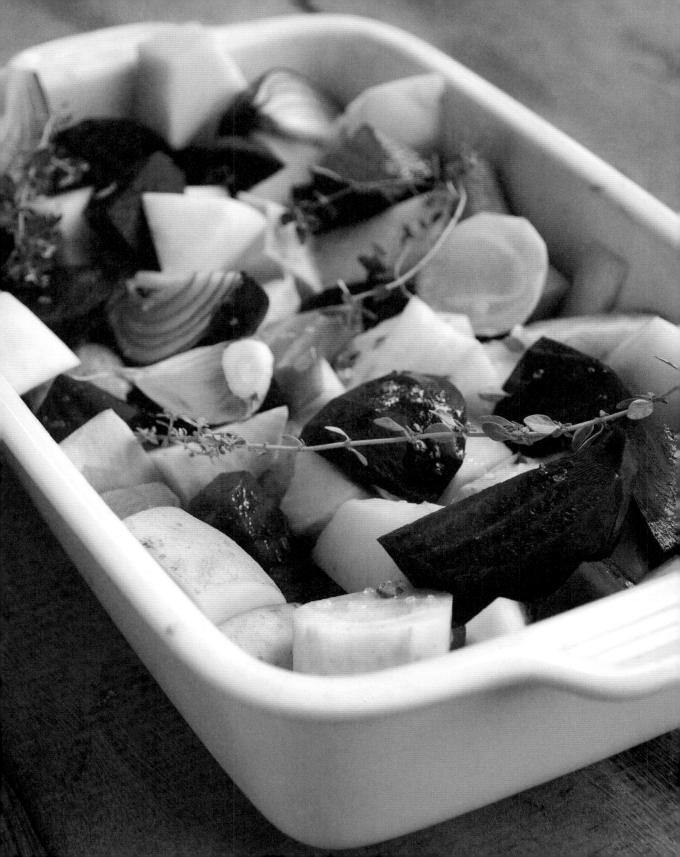

THAI VEGETABLE CURRY

PALEO-FRIENDLY VEGAN GLUTEN-FREE

SERVES 4 • PREP TIME: 15 MINUTES • COOK TIME: 45 MINUTES

Many types of vegetables work well with curry seasoning, so do not feel like you have to stick with the combination found in this recipe. Throw in squash, celeriac, bell peppers, zucchini, green beans, or whatever you have in the crisper of your refrigerator. If you use an assortment of veggies, you might have to stagger their addition to the dish so that the more delicate ones do not get overcooked.

1 tablespoon coconut oil

1 sweet onion, peeled and diced

2 teaspoons minced garlic

2 teaspoons grated fresh ginger

2 carrots, peeled and diced

1 sweet potato, peeled and diced

1 tablespoon curry powder

1 teaspoon ground cumin

2 cups vegetable broth

1 (28-ounce) can diced tomatoes with liquid

1 cup canned coconut milk

½ cup shredded coconut

2 cups finely julienned kale

1. Set a large pot over medium-high heat and add the coconut oil.

2. Sauté the onion, garlic, and ginger until softened, for 3 minutes.

3. Add the carrots and sweet potato and sauté for 6 more minutes, stirring often.

4. Add the curry powder, cumin, vegetable broth, diced tomatoes, and coconut milk and stir to mix well.

5. Bring the curry to a boil and then reduce the heat to low.

6. Simmer the curry until most of the sauce is thick and vegetables are tender, for 30 minutes.

7. Stir in the coconut and kale and simmer for an additional 5 minutes.

8. Serve plain or over rice.

TIP   No two curry powders in the store have the same flavor because curry is a spice mixture, not a single spice. The quantities of the different spices that go into curry can differ according to recipes, so try several mixes to get the one you like best. You can also mix up your own curry powder using cumin, coriander, turmeric, cloves, cayenne, paprika, and ginger.

QUINOA PUMPKIN STEW

VEGAN GLUTEN-FREE

SERVES 4 • PREP TIME: 15 MINUTES • COOK TIME: 40 MINUTES

If you do not have fresh pumpkin for this recipe, you can use canned pure pumpkin to get the same delightful flavor, although the texture will not be the same. Sweet potato or squash will also work, but try to use pumpkin if possible because it can actually boost your mood while you enjoy your meal. Pumpkin contains L-tryptophan, a feel-good amino acid.

---

1 tablespoon coconut oil

1 sweet onion, peeled and diced

2 teaspoons minced garlic

1 cup canned coconut milk

1 (15-ounce) can diced tomatoes, undrained

1 (15-ounce) can chickpeas, drained and rinsed

2 cups diced pumpkin (½-inch pieces)

2 cups cooked quinoa

Sea salt

Freshly ground black pepper

2 scallions, thinly sliced for garnish

1. Set a large saucepan over medium-high heat and add the coconut oil.
2. Sauté the onion and garlic in the oil until the vegetables are softened, for 3 minutes.
3. Add the coconut milk, tomatoes, chickpeas, and pumpkin.
4. Bring the liquid to a boil and then reduce the heat to low to simmer.
5. Simmer the stew until the pumpkin is tender, about 25 minutes.
6. Add the quinoa and stir to combine.
7. Simmer for an additional 3 minutes.
8. Season with salt and pepper.
9. Serve topped with scallions.

TIP Don't worry if you have a lot of extra pumpkin left over after making this stew—it freezes beautifully. Cut whatever is left into chunks, spread them out on a baking sheet, and freeze. When the pumpkin is frozen, transfer it to a sealable plastic bag and store in the freezer for up to 3 months.

VEGETABLE TOSS WITH COCONUT SAUCE

PALEO-FRIENDLY **VEGAN** GLUTEN-FREE

SERVES 4 • PREP TIME: 15 MINUTES • COOK TIME: 20 MINUTES

This meal can be on your table in just over 30 minutes, so try it on evenings when you have to run out the door for classes, sports, or social events. The starchy root vegetables are filling and help thicken the sauce, while the green beans and bell pepper enrich the flavor and add bright color to the dish. You can spoon your finished recipe over rice or couscous if you want to feed more than four people.

---

2 Yukon gold potatoes, peeled and cut into ¼-inch chunks

2 carrots, peeled and cut into ½-inch chunks

2 parsnips, peeled and cut into ½-inch chunks

½ head cauliflower, cut into florets

2 cups green beans, cut into 1-inch pieces

1 tablespoon coconut oil

½ sweet onion, diced

1 red pepper, diced

1 cup canned coconut milk

1 tablespoon maple syrup

1 teaspoon turmeric

Pinch cayenne pepper

Sea salt

¼ cup chopped fresh basil, for garnish

1. Set a large saucepan filled with water over medium-high heat and bring to a boil.

2. Add the potatoes, carrots, and parsnips and boil until tender, about 10 minutes.

3. Scoop the vegetables out into a bowl and set aside.

4. Add the cauliflower and green beans and boil until tender-crisp, about 4 minutes.

5. Drain and add to the bowl with the other vegetables. Set aside.

6. Set a large skillet over medium-high heat, add the coconut oil, and sauté the onion and red pepper until softened, for 3 minutes.

7. Stir in the coconut milk, maple syrup, turmeric, and cayenne pepper.

8. Stir to blend well, about 1 minute.

9. Season with salt.

10. Add the reserved vegetables and stir to combine.

11. Serve topped with the chopped basil.

SWEET POTATO–GINGER CASSEROLE

GLUTEN-FREE

SERVES 4 • PREP TIME: 15 MINUTES • COOK TIME: 30 MINUTES

Casseroles are a convenient way for busy people to get a nutritious meal with an array of yummy ingredients. Sweet potatoes, red lentils, earthy parsnips, and carrots, accented with toasty cumin, make a unique and filling dinner. Parsnips are high in potassium, folic acid, and fiber, which makes them effective for lowering cholesterol, regulating blood glucose levels, and reducing the risk of cardiovascular disease.

2 tablespoons coconut oil

1 sweet onion, peeled and chopped

2 teaspoons minced garlic

2 teaspoons grated fresh ginger

4 sweet potatoes, peeled and cut into ½-inch chunks

2 carrots, peeled and sliced

2 parsnips, peeled and sliced

1 teaspoon ground cumin

3 cups vegetable broth

1 cup canned coconut milk

2 cups dried red lentils

¼ cup sour cream for garnish

1. Preheat the oven to 375°F.
2. Set a large oven-proof skillet over medium-high heat and add the coconut oil.
3. Sauté the onion, garlic, and ginger until softened, for 3 minutes.
4. Add the sweet potatoes, carrots, and parsnips.
5. Sauté until the vegetables are golden brown, about 6 minutes.
6. Stir in the cumin, broth, coconut milk, and lentils and then bring the mixture to a boil.
7. Cover the skillet and put it in the oven until the lentils are tender and the sauce is thick, about 20 minutes.
8. Serve topped with sour cream.

TIP
You can use any color lentil for this recipe; they all promote a healthy heart, boost your energy, and help stabilize blood sugar. Lentils are high in fiber, protein, iron, and B vitamins and low in fat and calories.

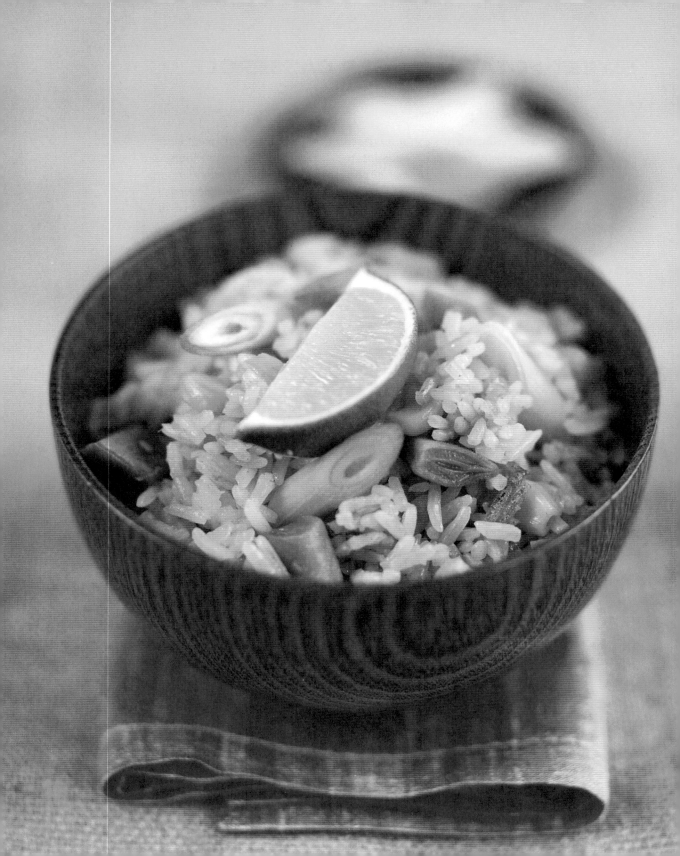

COCONUT-LIME RICE

PALEO-FRIENDLY VEGAN GLUTEN-FREE

SERVES 4 • PREP TIME: 20 MINUTES • COOK TIME: 30 MINUTES

Looking for a charming, simple dish bursting with fresh color and a hint of citrus? Try this rice creation for a light evening repast or a candlelit meal for a special someone. You need to keep the vegetables tender-crisp and the seasoning light for perfect execution of the dish. For a stronger citrus flavor, use 2 limes instead of 1 or add a splash of lemon juice right at the end of the preparation.

1 tablespoon coconut oil

2 teaspoons grated fresh ginger

1 teaspoon minced garlic

2 scallions, finely chopped

1 cup basmati rice

1 cup canned coconut milk

1 cup vegetable broth

½ teaspoon sea salt

2 cups blanched green beans, cut into ½-inch pieces

1 cup corn

Zest of 1 lime

Lime wedges, for garnish

1. Set a large saucepan over medium-high heat and add the coconut oil.

2. Sauté the ginger and garlic until the vegetables are softened, for 3 minutes.

3. Add the scallions and rice. Sauté for 2 minutes.

4. Stir in the coconut milk, vegetable broth, and salt.

5. Bring the liquid to a boil and then reduce the heat to low so that the rice simmers.

6. Simmer until the rice is tender, about 20 minutes.

7. Stir in the green beans, corn, and lime zest.

8. Let the rice sit for 5 minutes.

9. Serve topped with lime wedges.

COCONUT PAD THAI

GLUTEN-FREE

SERVES 6 • PREP TIME: 30 MINUTES PLUS CHILLING TIME • COOK TIME: 0 MINUTES

Coconut aminos might not be a familiar ingredient in your pantry, but it should be, because it is very high in vitamin C, potassium, and amino acids. Coconut aminos is made from coconut sap and tastes very similar to soy sauce. This ingredient is often used in Paleo dishes because it does not contain soy.

For the sauce

¼ cup peanut butter

¼ cup canned coconut milk

2 tablespoons coconut aminos

2 tablespoons honey

4 teaspoons minced garlic

1 tablespoon melted coconut oil

1 teaspoon minced chile

Pinch sea salt

For the vegetables

2 cups julienned fresh coconut

2 cups shredded napa cabbage

2 cups shredded carrot

½ sweet onion, very thinly sliced

2 scallions, sliced thinly

1 chile, finely chopped

½ cup chopped fresh cilantro

¼ cup shredded unsweetened coconut

To make the sauce

1. In a small bowl, whisk together the peanut butter, coconut milk, coconut aminos, honey, garlic, coconut oil, and chile until blended.

2. Season with salt and set aside.

To make the vegetables

1. In a large bowl, toss together the coconut, cabbage, carrot, onion, scallions, chile, cilantro, and coconut until evenly mixed.

2. Add the sauce to the vegetables and toss to combine.

3. Put the bowl in the refrigerator for 2 hours to let the flavors mellow.

4. Serve.

TIP Scallions are also called green onions, and they are not just a pretty addition to your recipes as a garnish. Scallions are an excellent source of antioxidants, as well as vitamins A, B, C, and K. These immature lily plants should be about as wide as a pencil and have snowy white bulbs and firm, vibrant green stalks in order to get the best flavor for your dish.

PEANUT-COCONUT NOODLES

VEGAN

SERVES 4 • PREP TIME: 15 MINUTES • COOK TIME: 15 MINUTES

Somen noodles cook very quickly because they are thin and stretched in production. They are usually served cold so that they do not get overcooked and mushy. You will be rinsing the noodle in this recipe so that they stay a pleasing texture and then serving them immediately after tossing with warm dressing and vegetables. For best results, keep the noodles separate from the other components of this dish until you are ready to serve.

For the sauce	For the noodles
2 cups canned coconut milk	2 (14-ounce) packages somen noodles
¾ cup peanut butter	2 tablespoons coconut oil
2 tablespoons grated fresh ginger	2 carrots, peeled and julienned
1 tablespoon minced garlic	2 red bell peppers, julienned
1 tablespoon coconut aminos	2 cups julienned bok choy
Juice from 1 lime	1 cup bean sprouts
Pinch red pepper flakes	2 scallions, julienned

To make the sauce

1. In a small saucepan over medium heat, whisk together the coconut milk, peanut butter, ginger, garlic, coconut aminos, lime juice, and red pepper flakes.

2. Bring the sauce to a boil, then reduce the heat to low and simmer for about 3 minutes.

3. Remove the sauce from the heat and set aside.

To make the noodles

1. Prepare the noodles according to package directions, rinse in cold water, and set aside.

2. Set a large skillet over medium-high heat and add the coconut oil.

3. Sauté the carrots, red peppers, bok choy, and sprouts until they are tender-crisp, about 8 minutes.

4. Add the scallions and noodles and sauté 2 more minutes.

5. Stir in the sauce and toss to coat the noodles.

6. Serve.

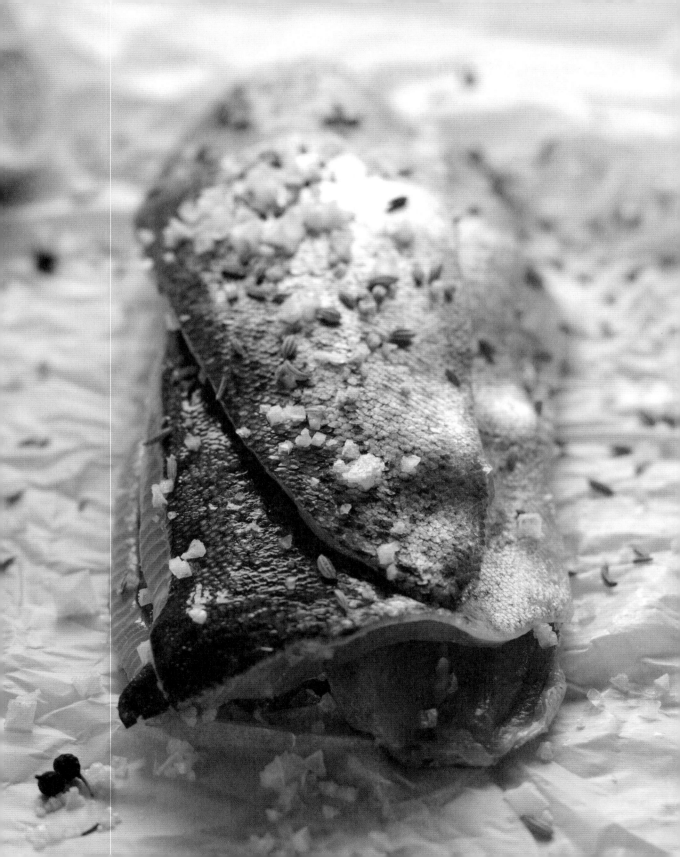

Chapter Eleven

FISH & SEAFOOD ENTRÉES

BAKED COCONUT SHRIMP WITH TANGERINE SALSA

PALEO-FRIENDLY GLUTEN-FREE

SERVES 4 • PREP TIME: 25 MINUTES • COOK TIME: 10 MINUTES

Shrimp is a bit of a touchy ingredient these days because much of the shrimp cultivated in open natural habitats is considered to be damaging to the environment, and farmed shrimp is poorer quality. There is sustainable shrimp available if you ask questions and look at product labels to see if the shellfish are endorsed by independent agencies such as the Marine Stewardship Council.

For the salsa

4 tangerines, peeled and chopped

1 lime, peeled and chopped

½ red bell pepper, finely chopped

1 teaspoon chopped fresh cilantro

1 teaspoon olive oil

Sea salt

Freshly ground black pepper

For the shrimp

Nonstick cooking spray to grease the baking sheet

½ cup almond flour

½ teaspoon garlic powder

2 eggs

1 cup shredded unsweetened coconut

1 pound (21–25 count) raw shrimp, peeled and deveined with the tails on

To make the salsa

1. In a small bowl, mix together the tangerines, lime, red pepper, cilantro, and oil.

2. Season with salt and pepper. Set aside.

To make the shrimp

1. Preheat the oven to 450°F.

2. Lightly coat a baking sheet with cooking spray. Set aside.

3. In a medium bowl, toss together the flour and garlic powder until well mixed and place the bowl on your work surface.

4. In a small bowl, whisk the eggs until well beaten and place this bowl beside the flour mixture.

5. Pour the coconut onto a plate and set the plate beside the eggs.

6. Dredge the shrimp in the flour mixture holding onto the tail, then dip the shrimp in the egg.

7. Shake off the extra egg and dredge the shrimp in the coconut.

8. Lay the coconut-crusted shrimp on the prepared baking sheet and repeat with the remaining shrimp.

9. Bake the shrimp until they are cooked through and the coconut is golden brown, about 10 minutes.

10. Serve the shrimp with the tangerine salsa.

TIP   Shrimp is very high in omega-3 fatty acids, protein, copper, selenium, vitamin B_{12}, phosphorus, and choline, which means shrimp can help reduce the risk of type 2 diabetes, cardiovascular disease, and depression. If you have high cholesterol, you might want to limit your shrimp intake, because a 4-ounce portion contains 220 milligrams of cholesterol.

COCONUT-SAFFRON SOUP

PALEO-FRIENDLY GLUTEN-FREE

SERVES 4 • PREP TIME: 20 MINUTES • COOK TIME: 15 MINUTES

You need very little saffron to create a dish with glorious flavor and lovely color. In order to achieve the best flavor, you need to ensure that you get real saffron rather than a cheaper substitute. Saffron is always expensive because it takes over 5,000 crocus flowers to produce 1 ounce of saffron from the flowers' stigmas. Your saffron threads should have a lighter tip than the rest of the thread; if you see saffron threads that are one solid color from end to end, then they are actually dyed stigmas from different flowers.

---

1 tablespoon coconut oil

2 teaspoons grated fresh ginger

2 teaspoons minced garlic

4 cups chicken broth

1 (15-ounce) can coconut milk

Juice of 1 lime

2 carrots, peeled and thinly sliced

2 cups snow peas, julienned

1 cup shredded kale

1 pound shrimp, peeled, deveined, and chopped

½ cup warm water

Pinch saffron threads

1 cup shredded coconut

Sea salt

2 scallions, chopped for garnish

1. Set a large saucepan over medium heat and add the coconut oil.

2. Sauté the ginger and garlic until softened, about 2 minutes.

3. Add the chicken broth, coconut milk, and lime juice.

4. Bring the soup to a boil and add the carrots, snow peas, kale, and shrimp.

5. Reduce the heat to low and simmer the soup until the shrimp is almost cooked through, about 5 minutes.

6. While the soup is simmering, put the saffron in warm water in a small bowl and let it sit.

7. Stir the saffron mixture and add to the soup with the coconut. Simmer 5 more minutes.

8. Season with salt and serve topped with scallions.

GOLDEN CRAB CAKES

PALEO-FRIENDLY GLUTEN-FREE

SERVES 3 • PREP TIME: 15 MINUTES PLUS CHILLING TIME • COOK TIME: 8 MINUTES

The sweetness of the crabmeat, hint of citrus, and chewy texture of coconut combine beautifully to create tender patties that can be served with an assortment of fruit salsas, sauces, or plain. These cakes can also be made ahead and frozen with absolutely no loss of quality. Simply take out the number you need and thaw completely before frying them up to a golden finish.

1 pound cooked lump crabmeat, drained and picked over

3 tablespoons shredded unsweetened coconut

1 tablespoon almond meal

1 tablespoon Dijon mustard

2 green onions, finely chopped

1 egg

1 teaspoon lemon zest

Pinch cayenne pepper

3 tablespoons coconut flour

1 tablespoon coconut oil

1. In a medium bowl, mix together the crabmeat, coconut, almond meal, Dijon mustard, green onions, egg, lemon zest, and cayenne pepper.

2. Divide the crab mixture into 9 patties about 1 inch thick. The cakes should hold together when pressed; if they don't, add more almond meal.

3. Chill the patties, covered, in the refrigerator for 1 hour or overnight to firm them up.

4. Spread the flour on a plate and dredge the chilled crab cakes in the flour until they are lightly coated.

5. Set a large skillet over medium heat and add the coconut oil.

6. Cook the crab cakes until they are golden, turning once, about 4 minutes per side.

7. Serve 3 patties per person.

TIP Good-quality crab is an ingredient that can be purchased conveniently in a can, because it can be very difficult to get the succulent flesh out of the legs and claws. Crab is an excellent source of protein, omega-3 fatty acids, selenium, and chromium. Include this luxurious ingredient in your diet to lower your risk of cancer and promote heart health.

MUSSELS IN HERBED COCONUT MILK

PALEO-FRIENDLY GLUTEN-FREE

SERVES 4 • PREP TIME: 15 MINUTES • COOK TIME: 15 MINUTES

You might think you are dining in a fancy restaurant when you serve up a steaming bowl of these exceptional mussels. Take the time to prepare your mussels correctly before cooking them, which means discarding mussels that are open, chipped, or broken. When you debeard your mussels, always pull the protruding byssal threads toward the hinge end, or you will kill the mussel.

2 tablespoons coconut oil

½ sweet onion, thinly sliced

1 teaspoon minced garlic

1 teaspoon grated fresh ginger

1 cup canned coconut milk

Juice of ½ lemon

1½ pounds fresh mussels, scrubbed and debearded

½ red bell pepper, minced

1 scallion, sliced thinly on a bias

1. Set a large saucepan over medium-high heat and add the coconut oil.

2. Sauté the onion, garlic, and ginger until softened, for 3 minutes.

3. Stir in the coconut milk and lemon juice to the skillet and bring to a boil.

4. Add the mussels, cover, and steam until the shells are open, about 8 minutes. Discard any unopened shells and take the skillet off the heat.

5. Stir in the red pepper and scallion.

6. Serve immediately with the sauce.

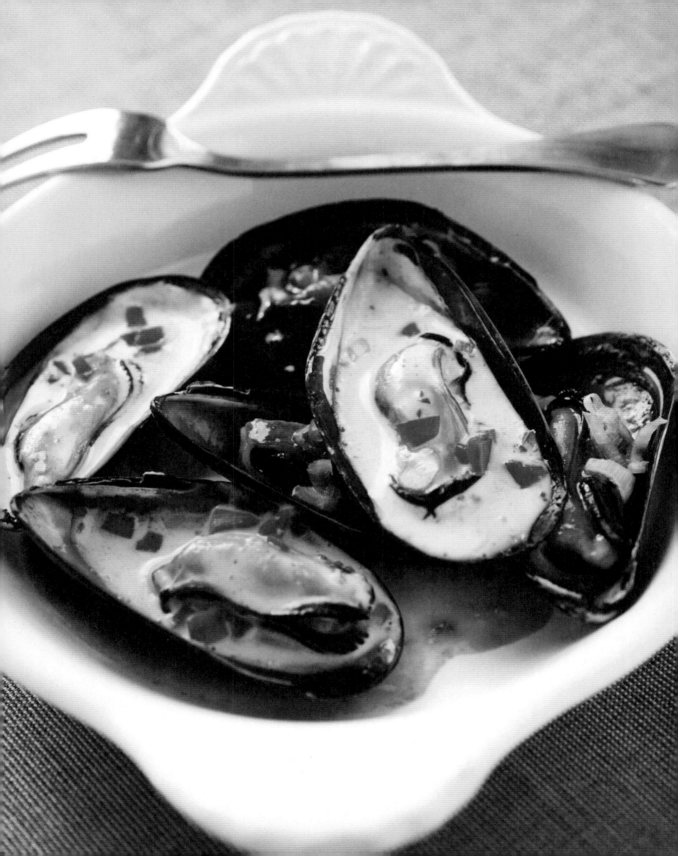

COCONUT SALMON CAKES

PALEO-FRIENDLY GLUTEN-FREE

SERVES 3 • PREP TIME: 15 MINUTES PLUS CHILLING TIME • COOK TIME: 8 MINUTES

Fresh salmon fillets can be used in this recipe instead of canned fish, but you will have to cook the fresh fish first and flake it so that the timing works. Coconut flour is used to bind these cakes together along with the egg, so if the mixture seems too wet when you try to form your cakes, add a little more coconut flour. Coconut flour is a tricky ingredient to use because it does not behave like regular flour. Coconut flour absorbs a great deal of liquid, so if you add too much your patties will fall apart.

1 (15-ounce) can salmon, drained

1 scallion, finely chopped

2 tablespoons coconut flour

1 teaspoon shredded unsweetened coconut

1 teaspoon grated fresh ginger

1 beaten egg

Juice of 1 lime

1 tablespoon chopped fresh parsley

Pinch sea salt

Pinch freshly ground black pepper

1 tablespoon coconut oil

1. In a large bowl, stir together the salmon, scallion, coconut flour, coconut, ginger, egg, lime juice, parsley, salt, and pepper until well mixed.

2. Form the salmon mixture into 9 equal patties, each 3 inches in diameter.

3. Chill the salmon patties in the refrigerator until firm, for 1 hour.

4. Set a large skillet over medium-high heat and add the coconut oil.

5. Cook the salmon patties, turning once, until lightly browned, about 4 minutes per side.

6. Serve 3 patties per person.

TILAPIA CURRY PACKETS

PALEO-FRIENDLY GLUTEN-FREE

SERVES 4 • PREP TIME: 20 MINUTES • COOK TIME: 20 MINUTES

Professional chefs can have difficulty cooking fish perfectly after years of practice, but cooking fish in packets, either parchment or foil, is a foolproof method of creating succulent, flaky fish every time. The packets keep all the juices and seasonings together, so take care when opening your packages so that you do not lose a single delicious drop.

---

1 large red bell pepper, seeded and thinly sliced into strips

2 cups small broccoli florets

1 cup bean sprouts

2 scallions, chopped

4 (5-ounce) tilapia fillets

1 cup canned coconut milk

2 teaspoons red curry paste

Juice of 1 lime

2 teaspoons grated fresh ginger

¼ cup shredded coconut

1. Preheat the oven to 400°F.

2. Cut 4 pieces of foil, each 12 inches square.

3. Evenly divide the red pepper, broccoli, bean sprouts, and scallions and put the vegetables onto the middle of each piece of foil.

4. Put a tilapia fillet on each pile of vegetables and turn up the edges of the foil a little to form bowls.

5. In a small bowl, whisk together the coconut milk, curry paste, lime juice, and ginger.

6. Pour the sauce evenly over the fish and sprinkle each piece with coconut.

7. Fold the foil up to form sealed packets and put them on a baking sheet.

8. Bake until the fish flakes when pressed with a fork, about 20 minutes.

9. Remove the tilapia and vegetables from the foil and serve.

TIP You can create packets out of parchment instead of foil if you want a more traditional preparation. Folding parchment tightly enough to form a packet that allows the fish to steam in its own juice can take some practice. Make sure you create sharp creases in the paper and fold the end edges under instead of up so the weight of the packet contents keeps the paper from undoing.

COCONUT-CRUSTED HALIBUT

PALEO-FRIENDLY GLUTEN-FREE

SERVES 4 • PREP TIME: 10 MINUTES PLUS CHILLING TIME • COOK TIME: 12 MINUTES

Fish is enhanced beautifully by nut crusts because the fat in the nut adds depth of flavor and richness to the milder fish flesh. Although not technically a nut, coconut makes a superb crust for fish. The addition of almond flour makes this dish gluten-free and Paleo friendly, but you can use regular flour if you are not following a special diet.

4 (5-ounce) boneless halibut fillets

Sea salt

Freshly ground black pepper

1 cup shredded unsweetened coconut

2 tablespoons almond flour

1 tablespoon coconut oil, melted

1. Preheat the oven to 400°F.

2. Line a baking sheet with parchment and set aside.

3. Pat the fillets dry with paper towels and lightly season the fish with salt and pepper.

4. In a small bowl, stir together the coconut and flour.

5. Press the halibut pieces in the coconut mixture so both sides of each piece are coated with coconut.

6. Put the fish on the baking sheet and drizzle with coconut oil.

7. Bake the fish in the oven until the topping is golden and the fish flakes easily with a fork, for 12 minutes total.

8. Serve.

TIP You might find it difficult to find sustainable fresh-caught halibut at grocery store fish counters. Ask in the store or at a favorite fishmonger where the fish came from and when it was caught to ensure quality and freshness. The best halibut comes from the Pacific Ocean produced in Canadian, Californian, and Alaskan fisheries.

COCONUT MILK–BRAISED COD

PALEO-FRIENDLY GLUTEN-FREE

SERVES 4 • PREP TIME: 15 MINUTES PLUS RESTING TIME • COOK TIME: 35 MINUTES

Baking proteins in liquid is an effective culinary technique to create a tender, flavorful meal. If the cod in this recipe was not baked first before adding the sauce, you would have been poaching your fish instead. Baking the cod cuts down on the cooking time and creates an appetizing brown color on the outside of the fish. This golden finish gives the dish a more attractive appearance.

---

2 pounds cod fillets

1 tablespoon freshly squeezed lemon juice

6 tablespoons coconut oil, divided

Sea salt

Freshly ground black pepper

1 sweet onion, chopped

2 teaspoons minced garlic

1 teaspoon minced jalapeño pepper

1 large tomato, chopped

½ teaspoon ground turmeric

¼ teaspoon sea salt

1 cup canned coconut milk

¼ cup chopped fresh cilantro, for garnish

1. Preheat the oven to 350°F.

2. Rub the cod fillets with lemon juice and 2 tablespoons coconut oil.

3. Season with salt and pepper and set the fish aside for 30 minutes.

4. Set a large skillet over medium-high heat and sauté the onion, garlic, and jalapeño until the vegetables are softened, about 3 minutes.

5. Add the tomato, turmeric, salt, and coconut milk. Stir to combine and bring to a boil.

6. Simmer the sauce for 5 minutes and remove the skillet from the heat.

7. Put the fish in a 9-by-9-inch baking dish and roast in the oven for 10 minutes.

8. Add the sauce to the baking dish, cover, and bake until the fish flakes with a fork, about 15 minutes.

9. Serve topped with cilantro.

TIP Tomatoes become more nutritious if they are cooked, because the levels of a phytonutrient called lycopene increase when the tomatoes are heated. Lycopene can help protect against heart disease and cancer. Tomatoes are also very high in fiber and vitamins A, C, and K.

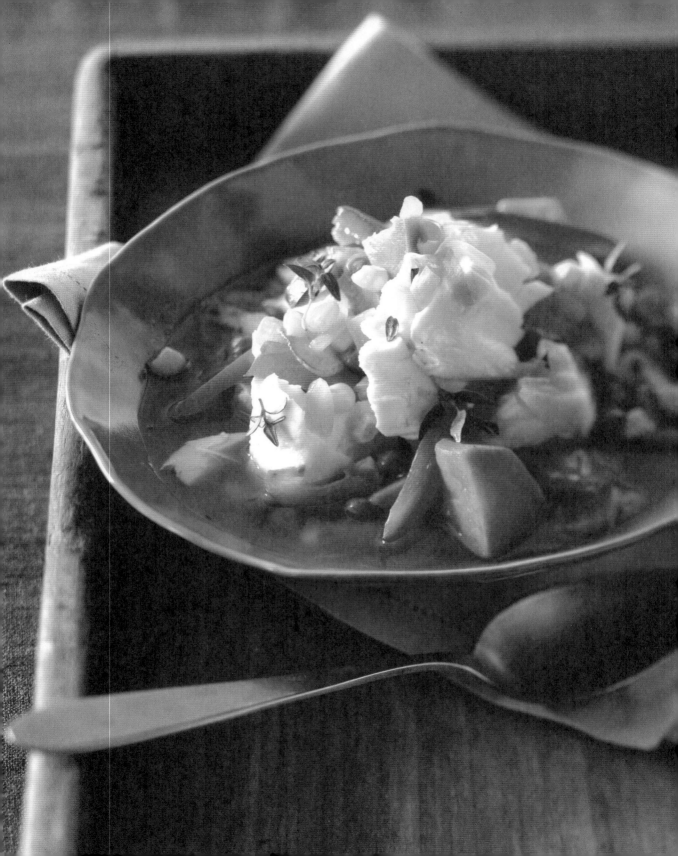

CARIBBEAN FISH STEW

PALEO-FRIENDLY GLUTEN-FREE

SERVES 4 • PREP TIME: 20 MINUTES • COOK TIME: 30 MINUTES

You might find a version of this flavorsome stew in Brazil, called Moqueca de Peixe. *Countries that have access to an abundance of fresh seafood often incorporate all kinds of fish and shellfish in one-pot meals designed to feed many people. This stew can be created with any combination of fish or shellfish, depending on what is fresh at your local store or favorite fishmonger. Do not compromise and use less than perfect fish, or the resulting product will be disappointing.*

2 tablespoons coconut oil

1 celery stalk, diced with greens

½ small onion, chopped

2 teaspoons minced garlic

2 teaspoons ground cumin

1 teaspoon paprika

5 cups vegetable broth

Juice of 2 limes

2 carrots, peeled and cut into 2-inch batons

1 sweet potato, peeled and cut into ½-inch chunks

16 ounces firm, white-fleshed fish, cubed

1 cup peas

1 cup corn

Pinch red pepper flakes

Sea salt

Freshly ground black pepper

1 teaspoon chopped fresh thyme

1. Set a large saucepan over medium-high heat and add the coconut oil.

2. Sauté the celery, onion, and garlic until the vegetables are softened, for 3 minutes.

3. Add the cumin and paprika and sauté an additional 1 minute.

4. Add the vegetable broth and lime juice and stir to combine.

5. Bring the stew to a boil and add the carrots and sweet potato.

6. Reduce the heat to low, cover, and simmer until the vegetables are almost tender, about 10 minutes.

7. Add the fish, peas, and corn and simmer 10 minutes more until the fish is tender.

8. Stir in the red pepper flakes and season with salt and pepper.

9. Serve the stew immediately, topped with the thyme.

BAKED SALMON WITH COCONUT BASMATI RICE

GLUTEN-FREE

SERVES 4 • PREP TIME: 15 MINUTES • COOK TIME: 25 MINUTES

Baking fish in a tasty bed of seasoned vegetables is a wonderful culinary method to infuse spectacular flavor and moisture into the fish. Spinach is a natural choice for pairing with salmon because the color combination is spectacular, and the earthy flavor of the greens does not overpower the assertive salmon. You can also use kale or Swiss chard with lovely results.

For the rice

1 cup basmati rice

1½ cups canned coconut milk

½ cup water

¼ teaspoon ground cinnamon

Pinch sea salt

For the salmon

6 cups spinach

1 red pepper, chopped

½ cup shredded unsweetened coconut

2 tablespoons melted coconut oil, divided

4 (6-ounce) salmon fillets

Sea salt

Freshly ground black pepper

To make the rice

1. Set a medium saucepan over medium heat and add the rice, coconut milk, water, cinnamon, and salt.

2. Bring the rice to a boil, reduce the heat to low, cover, and simmer until the rice is tender, about 20 minutes.

3. Remove from the heat and set aside.

To make the salmon

1. Preheat the oven to 400°F.

2. While the rice is cooking, in a large bowl, toss together the spinach, red pepper, coconut, and 1 tablespoon of the coconut oil.

3. Transfer the spinach mixture to a 9-by-13-inch baking dish and spread it out evenly.

4. Season the salmon lightly with salt and pepper.

5. Top the spinach mixture with the salmon fillets and drizzle the fish with the remaining tablespoon of oil.

6. Bake the salmon and spinach mixture until the fish flakes easily with a fork, about 15 minutes.

7. Serve the salmon and spinach over the coconut rice.

TIP Salmon is considered to be a very important addition to a nutritious diet because this fish is an excellent source of omega-3 fatty acids. Omega-3s decrease inflammation in the body, reduce the risk of cardiovascular disease, and promote brain and nerve health.

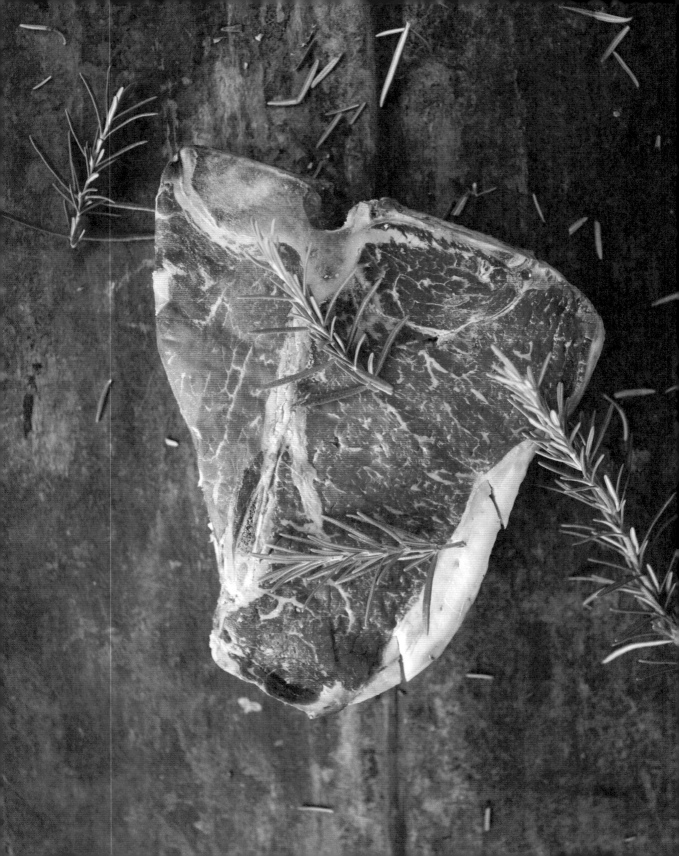

Chapter Twelve

POULTRY & MEAT ENTRÉES

COCONUT-LIME CHICKEN

PALEO-FRIENDLY GLUTEN-FREE

SERVES 4 • PREP TIME: 20 MINUTES PLUS CHILLING TIME • COOK TIME: 20 MINUTES

Chicken fingers do not just have to be for kids; this adult version breads the chicken breast with shredded coconut and finely ground almonds. The dipping sauce is sweet and made complex with salty coconut aminos and tart lime zest. The sauce can be made the day before and stored in the refrigerator in a sealed container until you want to use it for your chicken strips.

For the sauce

1 cup canned coconut milk

Juice and zest from 1 lime

1 tablespoon honey

1 teaspoon minced garlic

1 teaspoon coconut aminos

For the chicken

¾ cup almond flour

2 eggs, beaten

¾ cup shredded unsweetened coconut

½ cup ground almonds

¼ teaspoon ground nutmeg

¼ teaspoon sea salt

4 (5-ounce) boneless, skinless chicken breasts, cut into 4 strips each

3 tablespoons coconut oil, melted

To make the sauce

1. Set a small saucepan over medium heat and add the coconut milk, lime juice and zest, honey, garlic, and coconut aminos.

2. Bring to a boil and then reduce the heat to low and simmer for 5 minutes to thicken and mellow the flavor.

3. Remove from the heat and pour into a bowl. Chill in the refrigerator for 2 hours.

To make the chicken

1. Preheat the oven to 350°F.

2. Line a baking sheet with parchment paper and set aside.

3. Put the flour in a bowl and place the bowl on your work surface.

4. Put the beaten eggs in a bowl beside the flour.

5. In a medium bowl, stir together the coconut, ground almonds, nutmeg, and salt until well mixed. Put the coconut mixture beside the eggs.

6. Pat the chicken strips dry with paper towels and dredge each strip in the flour, then the egg mixture, and finally the coconut mixture to coat.

7. Put the breaded strips on the baking sheet.

8. Brush the strips carefully with the melted coconut oil.

9. Bake the chicken strips until golden brown and cooked through, turning once, about 12 minutes in total.

10. Serve with the lime dipping sauce.

TIP One 4-ounce portion of chicken breast provides 70 percent of the daily recommended amount of protein. This popular poultry is also extremely high in selenium, which can help reduce the risk of cancer and boost your immune system.

COCONUT CHICKEN NOODLE SALAD

GLUTEN-FREE

SERVES 4 • PREP TIME: 20 MINUTES PLUS CHILLING TIME • COOK TIME: 5 MINUTES

Rice noodles are gluten-free and can be cooked by soaking them for a few minutes in very hot liquid. Do not overcook the rice noodles because they will soak up the dressing when you toss all the ingredients together.

For the dressing
½ cup canned coconut milk
Juice of 2 limes
Zest of 1 lime
1 tablespoon honey
1 teaspoon fish sauce
½ teaspoon minced garlic
3 tablespoons melted coconut oil

For the noodles
2 cups water
2 cups canned coconut milk

4 ounces rice noodles
4 (5-ounce) cooked skinless chicken breasts, shredded
1 English cucumber, cut into long ribbons
1 red pepper, julienned
1 carrot, peeled and julienned
1 cup bean sprouts
1 jalapeño pepper, seeded and minced
¼ cup chopped peanuts
2 tablespoons chopped mint, for garnish

To make the dressing

In a small bowl, whisk together the coconut milk, lime juice, lime zest, honey, fish sauce, and garlic until well blended. Drizzle in the coconut oil and whisk to incorporate. Set the dressing aside.

To make the noodles

1. In a large saucepan over medium-high heat, combine the water and coconut milk and bring the mixture to a boil.

2. Place the noodles in a large bowl and pour the boiling coconut milk mixture over the noodles.

3. Stir the noodles and let them sit until they are cooked al dente, about 5 minutes.

4. Drain and pour the noodles into a large bowl and add the dressing.

5. Toss to combine, then add the chicken, cucumber, red pepper, carrot, bean sprouts, jalapeño, and peanuts and toss again, using tongs.

6. Cover the salad and put it in the refrigerator to chill, about 1 hour.

7. Toss with tongs again to mix, and serve the salad topped with the mint.

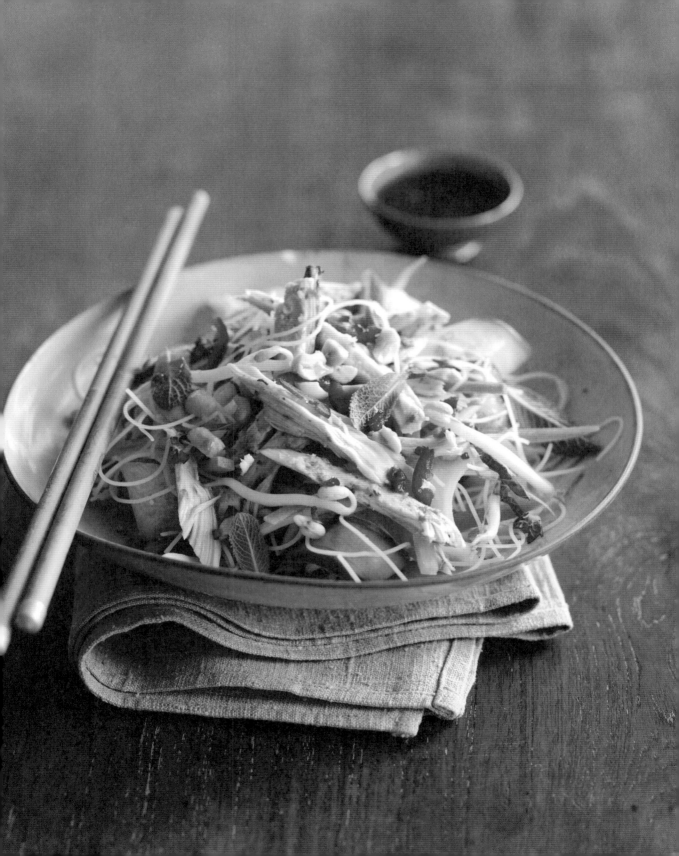

CHILI-GLAZED CHICKEN

PALEO-FRIENDLY GLUTEN-FREE

SERVES 4 • PREP TIME: 15 MINUTES PLUS MARINATING TIME • COOK TIME: 30 MINUTES

Barbecuing is a marvelous cooking technique for chicken, especially if the poultry still has the skin on it. If you do not have a barbecue or the weather is not conducive to standing outside, you can broil or roast the chicken as well. The cooking time will be a little longer, so make sure you cook your chicken to an internal temperature of 165°F.

For the glaze
½ cup rice vinegar
6 tablespoons honey
2 tablespoons coconut aminos
½ teaspoon red pepper flakes

For the chicken
4 (5-ounce) boneless chicken breasts
¼ cup canned coconut milk, at room temperature
2 teaspoons grated fresh ginger
1 teaspoon melted coconut oil
½ teaspoon red pepper flakes
3 scallions, thinly sliced, for garnish

To make the glaze

1. Set a small saucepan over medium heat and add the vinegar, honey, coconut aminos, and red pepper flakes.

2. Bring the mixture to a boil and reduce the heat to low and simmer, stirring constantly, until the liquid is reduced by half, about 6 minutes.

3. Set aside and cover to keep the glaze warm until the chicken is ready.

To make the chicken

1. Rinse the chicken and pat the breasts dry with paper towels. Cut the chicken lengthwise through the middle so that the chicken breast fans out without cutting the breast in half.

2. In a large bowl, stir together the coconut milk, ginger, coconut oil, and red pepper flakes.

3. Add the chicken breasts, turning to coat, then cover the bowl and refrigerate for 2 hours.

4. Preheat a barbecue to medium-high heat.

5. Take the chicken out of the bowl, and grill it, turning at least once, until the chicken is cooked through, for 20 minutes in total.

6. Transfer the breasts to a plate and drizzle the glaze over the meat evenly.

7. Garnish with the scallions and serve.

GRILLED ORANGE-COCONUT CHICKEN

PALEO-FRIENDLY GLUTEN-FREE

SERVES 6 • PREP TIME: 15 MINUTES PLUS MARINATING TIME • COOK TIME: 20 MINUTES

Oranges make for an agreeable marinade ingredient for this chicken because the sweetness merges with the pungent garlic and fresh thyme to create a classic flavor. Thyme is a delicate herb that contains many powerful antioxidants, including an impressive amount of vitamin C. Thyme is also an antimicrobial, which means it can ensure your marinated meat is safe to eat without any contamination.

---

4 chicken legs, cut into thighs and drumsticks

1 (15-ounce) can coconut milk

Juice of 2 oranges

¼ cup melted coconut oil

¼ cup chopped fresh thyme

3 teaspoons minced garlic

½ teaspoon sea salt

Orange wedges for garnish

1. Pierce the chicken pieces all over with a fork and transfer them to a large sealable plastic bag.

2. In a medium bowl, whisk together the coconut milk, orange juice, coconut oil, thyme, garlic, and salt.

3. Pour the marinade into the bag with the chicken and press out as much air as possible.

4. Seal the bag and turn to coat the chicken thoroughly with the marinade.

5. Put the bag in the refrigerator and let sit for 4 hours or overnight, turning at least once.

6. Preheat a barbecue to medium-high heat.

7. Remove the chicken from the bag and grill it, turning at least once, until the chicken is cooked through and golden, about 20 minutes.

8. Serve with orange wedges.

INDONESIAN CHICKEN SATAY

GLUTEN-FREE

SERVES 6 • PREP TIME: 10 MINUTES PLUS MARINATING TIME • COOK TIME: 10 MINUTES

Satay is another word for kebabs without the chunks of vegetables. You might find threading marinated chicken strips onto the wood skewers a bit messy, but the end product is worth the mess. It is important to soak the wood skewers in water for at least 30 minutes so that the skewers do not burn and break. You can also use metal skewers, but the presentation is not as traditional when you arrange the meat around a bowl of dipping sauce.

2 pounds boneless, skinless chicken breast, cut into strips

Juice of 2 limes

2 tablespoons melted coconut oil

2 tablespoons brown sugar

1 tablespoon finely chopped fresh cilantro

1 tablespoon minced garlic

1. Put the chicken strips in a large bowl and add the lime juice, coconut oil, brown sugar, cilantro, and garlic, tossing to coat the chicken.

2. Put the chicken, covered, in the refrigerator for 1 hour to marinate.

3. Remove the chicken from the marinade and thread the strips onto wooden skewers that have been soaked in water. Set aside on a plate.

4. Preheat the oven to Broil and lay each chicken satay skewer on a baking sheet lined with foil.

5. Broil the satay until cooked through and golden, 4 minutes per side.

6. Serve with your favorite dipping sauce.

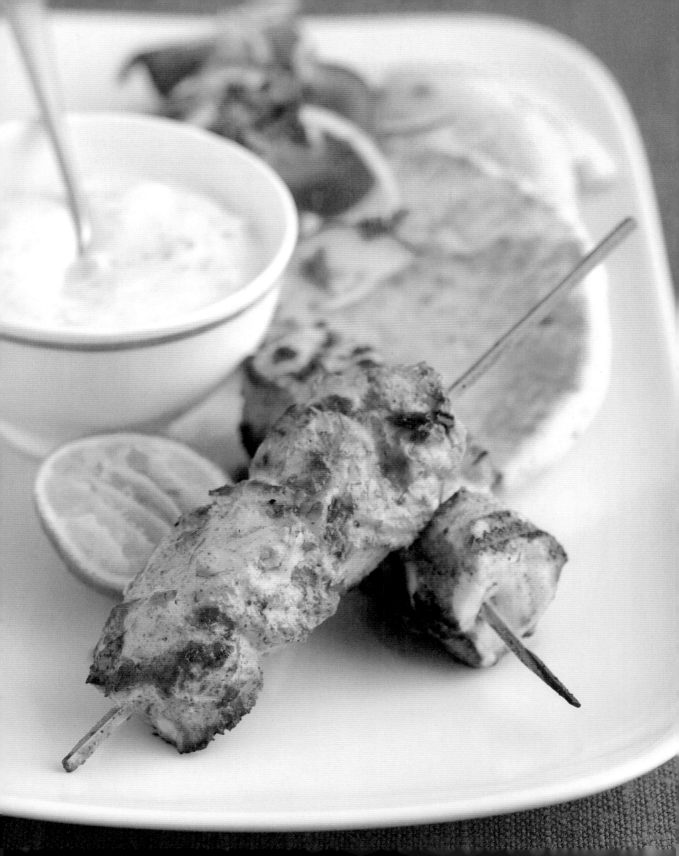

ROASTED COCONUT-LEMON CHICKEN

PALEO-FRIENDLY GLUTEN-FREE

SERVES 6 • PREP TIME: 10 MINUTES • COOK TIME: 1 HOUR 30 MINUTES

What is more family friendly than a golden roasted chicken set proudly on the table for Sunday dinner? Roasted chicken combines juicy meat with crispy flavorful skin, so you might not have much left over after the meal. This lack of extra chicken is a shame—having cooked chicken available can be incredibly convenient—so why not roast two chickens instead of one when making this recipe? When the chickens are ready, eat one for dinner and let the other bird cool down so you can strip off the meat and store it in sealable plastic bags in the refrigerator or freezer.

1 (4-pound) whole roasting chicken

1 teaspoon sea salt, divided

2 lemons, quartered

2 garlic cloves, lightly smashed

2 tablespoons melted coconut oil

1. Preheat the oven to 350°F.
2. Wash the chicken inside and out in cold water and pat it completely dry with paper towels.
3. Salt the cavity of the chicken with ½ teaspoon salt and stuff the cavity with the lemons and garlic.
4. Put the chicken in a large baking dish and brush the skin generously with the coconut oil.
5. Salt the chicken skin with the remaining salt.
6. Roast the chicken until it is golden brown and cooked through (an internal temperature of 185°F), about 1 hour and 30 minutes.
7. Remove the chicken from the oven and let it rest for about 15 minutes.
8. Remove the lemon and garlic.
9. Serve.

SIMPLE CHICKEN COCONUT CURRY

GLUTEN-FREE

SERVES 4 • PREP TIME: 15 MINUTES • COOK TIME: 45 MINUTES

Curry does not have to be complicated to be good. Simple lean chicken breast, a few potatoes, and the perfect balance of spices in a creamy coconut sauce makes for a pleasurable meal. If possible, make this recipe the day before you need it so that the flavors can blend and mellow. Reheat the curry over low heat as you cook a pot of fragrant basmati rice as an accompaniment.

---

1 tablespoon coconut oil

4 (5-ounce) boneless, skinless chicken breasts, cut into 1-inch chunks

1 tablespoon minced fresh garlic

1 tablespoon grated fresh ginger

2 cups chicken broth

2 cups canned coconut milk

2 potatoes, peeled and diced into ½-inch chunks

2 carrots, peeled and chopped

1 tablespoon good-quality curry powder

1 teaspoon ground cumin

½ teaspoon turmeric

¼ teaspoon sea salt

1. Set a large saucepan over medium-high heat and add the coconut oil.

2. Sauté the chicken breast until it is lightly browned and almost cooked through, about 7 minutes.

3. Remove the chicken with a slotted spoon and set aside in a bowl.

4. To the saucepan, add the garlic and ginger and sauté for 3 minutes.

5. Add the chicken broth, coconut milk, potatoes, carrots, curry, cumin, turmeric, salt, and reserved chicken to the pan.

6. Bring the curry to a boil, then reduce the heat to low and simmer.

7. Simmer until the vegetables and chicken are tender, about 30 minutes.

8. Serve over rice.

TIP Garlic has been an important element in herbal and natural medicine for centuries, especially to clean the blood and bolster the immune system. Garlic is a powerful antioxidant and antibiotic and can help protect the body from the free radicals that cause diseases such as cancer and cardiovascular disease.

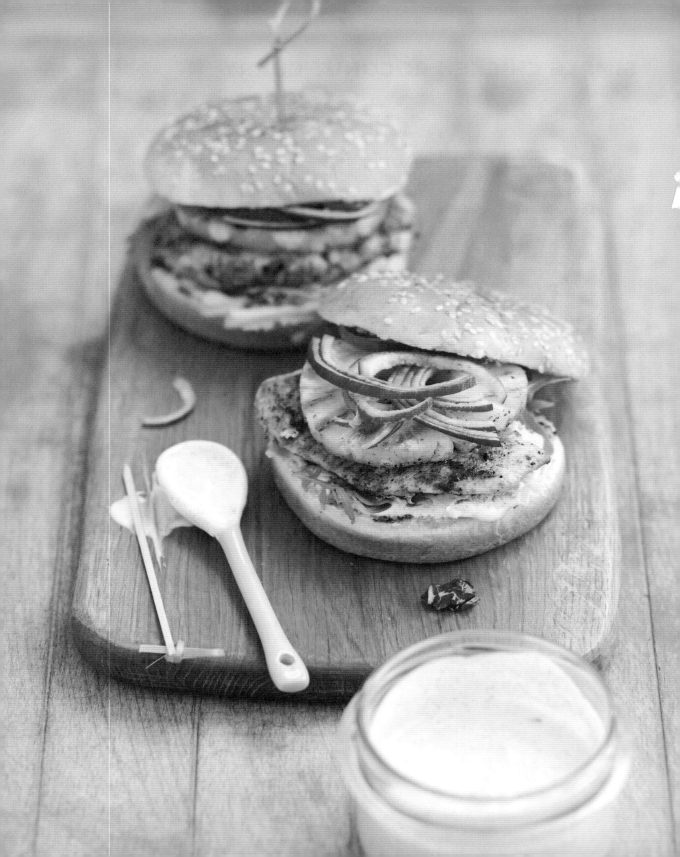

COCONUT CHICKEN BURGERS

SERVES 4 • PREP TIME: 20 MINUTES • COOK TIME: 20 MINUTES

Chicken burgers make a nice change from the usual beef choice, especially if you use quality lean chicken breast, grilled to perfection. The coconut mayonnaise is a lovely base for many types of toppings. Add a little roasted garlic, chopped tomato, or a touch of jalapeño pepper for interesting variations. You can serve this dish without the buns if you want a Paleo-friendly and gluten-free meal.

For coconut mayonnaise

2 large egg yolks

1½ tablespoons freshly squeezed lemon juice

1 teaspoon Dijon mustard

½ cup melted coconut oil

⅓ cup olive oil

Sea salt

Freshly ground black pepper

For chicken burgers

4 (4-ounce) skinless chicken breasts

1 tablespoon melted coconut oil

Sea salt

Freshly ground black pepper

1 cup arugula

4 slices fresh pineapple, about ½ inch thick

½ red onion, cut into 4 slices

4 sesame hamburger buns

To make the coconut mayonnaise

1. In a medium bowl, whisk together the egg yolks, lemon juice, and Dijon until smooth.

2. Keep whisking and slowly add the coconut oil in a thin stream to create a thick emulsion.

3. Continue whisking while adding the olive oil in a thin stream until all the oil is used up and the mayonnaise is thick.

4. Season with salt and pepper and adjust the taste with more lemon juice, if desired.

5. Keep the mayonnaise in a sealed container in the refrigerator for up to 1 week.

continued

To make the chicken burgers

1. Preheat a barbecue to medium-high heat.

2. Lightly brush the chicken breasts with coconut oil and season with salt and pepper.

3. Grill the chicken breasts until cooked through, turning once, about 7 minutes per side.

4. Grill the pineapple slices on a separate part of the barbecue, turning once, until lightly caramelized, about 2 minutes per side.

5. Spread the bottom half of each hamburger bun with coconut mayonnaise and top with ¼ cup of arugula.

6. Top the greens with a chicken breast, a slice of pineapple, red onion, and the top half of the bun.

7. Serve.

RED WINE VENISON STEW

PALEO-FRIENDLY GLUTEN-FREE

SERVES 6 • PREP TIME: 20 MINUTES • COOK TIME: 2 HOURS 15 MINUTES

Venison benefits from browning in coconut oil because it is a very lean meat that can dry out easily and become tough. Venison contains all the essential amino acids, making it a complete protein and healthful addition to any diet. Many people who follow the Paleo diet enjoy venison because the animals are usually allowed to roam around freely in fields, which makes them pasture raised.

---

2 tablespoons coconut oil

1 pound venison, cut into ½-inch chunks

1 sweet onion, chopped

3 teaspoons minced garlic

4 cups beef broth

1 cup dry red wine

8 tablespoons tomato paste

1 teaspoon smoked paprika

½ teaspoon dried marjoram

2 potatoes, peeled and diced large

2 carrots, peeled and sliced into ¼-inch-thick rounds

2 cups green beans, cut into 1-inch pieces

Sea salt

Freshly ground black pepper

1. Set a large stockpot over medium-high heat and add the coconut oil.

2. Brown the venison, about 6 minutes, and then use a slotted spoon to transfer the meat to a plate. Set aside.

3. Add the onion and garlic to the pot and sauté until softened, about 4 minutes.

4. Stir in the beef broth, red wine, tomato paste, paprika, marjoram, potatoes, carrots, and the reserved meat with accumulated juices from the plate.

5. Bring the stew to a boil and then reduce the heat to low and simmer until the venison is tender and the stew has thickened, about 2 hours.

6. Stir in the green beans and simmer until the beans are tender-crisp, about 5 minutes.

7. Season with salt and pepper, and serve.

TIP People used to consider potatoes poisonous, and this assumption was right to some extent. Potatoes contain a natural toxin called solanine that can make you sick and can in rare cases be fatal when consumed. Higher concentrations of this toxin will be found in potatoes that are greenish or have green eyes or sprouts. Throw these spuds away when you find them in your pantry.

ASIAN BEEF & PORK MEATBALLS

PALEO-FRIENDLY GLUTEN-FREE

SERVES 6 • PREP TIME: 20 MINUTES • COOK TIME: 20 MINUTES

Baking meatballs creates a tasty browned crust on the meat that is palate pleasing, but you can also braise these meatballs in a sauce or drop them into a simmering soup. If you like to batch cook, double this recipe and freeze the raw meatballs on a baking sheet before transferring them to sealable plastic bags for future use. Thaw the meatballs in the refrigerator before cooking them using your favorite technique.

Coconut oil for greasing the baking sheet

1 pound lean ground beef

1 pound ground pork

1 cup almond meal

1 egg

1 scallion, minced

¼ cup canned coconut milk

¼ cup shredded unsweetened coconut

2 tablespoons coconut aminos

1½ tablespoons minced garlic

1 tablespoon grated fresh ginger

Pinch sea salt

Pinch red pepper flakes

1. Preheat the oven to 400°F.

2. Lightly oil a baking sheet with coconut oil. Set aside.

3. In a large bowl, mix together the beef, pork, almond meal, egg, scallion, coconut milk, coconut, coconut aminos, garlic, ginger, salt, and red pepper flakes using your hands until very well combined.

4. Shape the beef mixture into 1½-inch balls and place them in a single layer on the baking sheet.

5. Bake the meatballs until they are cooked through, turning once, about 20 minutes.

6. Serve the meatballs on rice or as a tasty pita pocket filling.

TIP Meatballs freeze very well because they have a nice ratio of meat and fat that keeps them moist. You can use lamb or veal meat as well for a nice change of taste.

FIERY FRIED BEEF

PALEO-FRIENDLY GLUTEN-FREE

SERVES 6 • PREP TIME: 15 MINUTES PLUS MARINATING TIME • COOK TIME: 1 HOUR 50 MINUTES

This dish is mouth-scorching hot with a complexity of heat that is created by the habanero peppers and chili powder. The beef is not coated in sauce because the flavors and spices are cooked right into the meat. You can enjoy this dish by itself, but eating it with plain rice or piled on a crusty bun is the best method to highlight the taste of the beef.

4 teaspoons minced garlic

2 shallots, peeled and minced

2 teaspoons grated fresh ginger

2 teaspoons ground cinnamon

1 teaspoon chili powder

1 teaspoon ground coriander

½ teaspoon ground cumin

½ teaspoon ground cloves

½ teaspoon turmeric

2 pounds beef chuck, trimmed, and cut into 1-inch chunks

1 cup beef stock

¼ cup coconut oil

1 sweet onion, peeled and thinly sliced

1 habanero chile, minced

Juice of 2 limes

1 cup shredded unsweetened coconut

1. In a large sealable plastic bag, combine the garlic, shallots, ginger, cinnamon, chili powder, coriander, cumin, cloves, and turmeric. Using your fingers on the outside of the bag, form the spices and seasonings into a paste.

2. Add the beef and massage the bag to coat the meat with the paste.

3. Squeeze out as much air as possible and seal the bag. Put the bag in the refrigerator to marinate for 4 hours.

4. Set a large saucepan with a lid on high heat and bring the beef stock to a boil.

5. Add the beef chunks and any paste left in the bag to the broth, cover, reduce the heat to medium-low, and simmer until very tender, about 1½ hours. Remove the beef from the saucepan with a slotted spoon to a plate and set aside.

6. Set a large skillet over medium heat and melt the coconut oil.

7. Sauté the onion until lightly caramelized, about 8 minutes.

8. Add the chile and lime juice and sauté 2 more minutes.

9. Stir in the reserved beef and the coconut and sauté for 10 more minutes until the beef is lightly browned and any liquid in the skillet has evaporated.

10. Serve the beef over rice.

JUICY BEEF & PORK HAMBURGERS

SERVES 4 • PREP TIME: 10 MINUTES • COOK TIME: 15 MINUTES

Hamburger recipes are sometimes closely guarded secrets, and the quest for the perfect hamburger is the goal of TV cooking shows and contests all over North America. Some purists only use beef, and other burger experts feel a combination of proteins is the way to create the best. This recipe mixes beef and pork together with simple seasoning and very few other ingredients. You can grill these juicy patties on a barbecue, but pan searing them in coconut oil creates a tantalizing golden crust, sealing in the juices and flavor.

3 tablespoons coconut oil, divided

½ cup chopped sweet onion

1 teaspoon minced fresh garlic

1 pound lean ground beef

½ pound lean ground pork

1 egg

1 teaspoon chopped fresh thyme

Dash sea salt

Hamburger buns (optional)

1. Set a small skillet over medium heat. Add 1 tablespoon of coconut oil and sauté the onion and garlic until softened, for 3 minutes.

2. In a large bowl, mix together the ground beef, ground pork, egg, thyme, salt, and cooked vegetables.

3. Divide the meat mixture into 4 equal pieces and form into ½-inch-thick patties.

4. Set a large skillet over medium-high heat and add the remaining 2 tablespoons of coconut oil.

5. Pan sear the burgers for 4 to 5 minutes per side, or until they have reached your desired doneness.

6. Serve on a bun or as is.

CUMIN BEEF & PEPPERS

PALEO-FRIENDLY GLUTEN-FREE

SERVES 6 • PREP TIME: 25 MINUTES • COOK TIME: 2 HOURS

Tender beef chunks and lightly caramelized bell peppers are combined with an intense spicy sauce. If using a slow cooker, sauté the peppers separately before adding them to the finished dish.

---

3 tablespoons coconut oil, divided

1 pound beef chuck, trimmed and cut into 1-inch chunks

1 sweet onion, peeled and cut into eighths

2 teaspoons minced garlic

2 teaspoons grated fresh ginger

1 tablespoon ground cumin

¼ teaspoon ground coriander

½ teaspoon sea salt

¼ teaspoon cayenne pepper

Pinch allspice

1 cup canned coconut milk

½ cup beef stock

2 red bell peppers, cut into strips

1 yellow bell pepper, cut into strips

¼ cup chopped fresh cilantro

1. Preheat the oven to 325°F.

2. Set a large ovenproof skillet over medium-high heat and add 2 tablespoons of the coconut oil.

3. Brown the beef on all sides and remove the meat to a plate with a slotted spoon.

4. Add the onion to the skillet and sauté until it is soft, stirring frequently, about 5 minutes.

5. Add the garlic and ginger and sauté an additional 2 minutes.

6. Add the cumin, coriander, sea salt, cayenne pepper, and allspice and sauté 2 minutes.

7. Add the coconut milk, beef stock, and beef with accumulated juices from the plate. Stir to combine and bring the liquid to a boil, then cover the skillet and transfer it to the oven.

8. Braise the beef, stirring several times, until the meat is very tender, about 1½ hours.

9. Remove the skillet from the oven and set aside.

10. Set a small skillet over medium heat and add the remaining 1 tablespoon of coconut oil.

11. Sauté the peppers until they are tender and lightly browned, about 5 minutes.

12. Add the peppers to the beef mixture and serve over rice. Top with chopped cilantro.

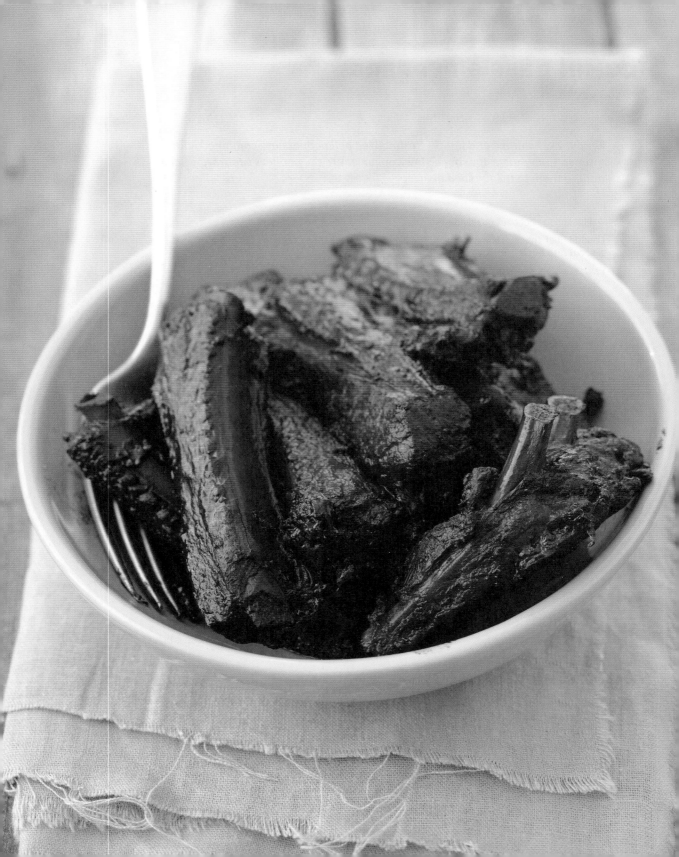

STICKY COCONUT PORK RIBS

GLUTEN-FREE

SERVES 6 • PREP TIME: 10 MINUTES PLUS MARINATING TIME • COOK TIME: 55 MINUTES

Braising your ribs before grilling or broiling them ensures tender, fall-off-the-bone results without overcooking the meat. The reason is that the brown sugar in the rib sauce can burn if placed near heat for too long, so braising makes sure that the meat is cooked without the sauce burning. The finished ribs are tender, sticky, and have a subtle Asian flavor from the ginger and coconut aminos.

---

4 pounds baby back pork ribs

2 cups chicken broth

1 (15-ounce) can coconut milk

4 garlic cloves

1 (2-inch) piece of peeled fresh ginger, chopped

½ cup chopped sweet onion

½ cup packed brown sugar

½ cup chopped fresh cilantro

¼ cup coconut aminos

½ teaspoon sea salt

1. Preheat the oven to 400°F.

2. Arrange the ribs in a large baking dish in one layer.

3. Add the chicken broth and enough water to cover the ribs by 1 inch.

4. Cover the baking dish tightly with foil and put in the oven.

5. Braise the ribs until they are tender but not falling off the bone, for about 45 minutes.

6. Remove the ribs from the oven and pour off the remaining liquid. Set aside.

7. Pour the coconut milk into a blender and add the garlic, ginger, onion, brown sugar, cilantro, coconut aminos, and salt.

8. Blend until the mixture is smooth.

9. Pour the coconut milk marinade over the ribs, turning them to ensure coverage, then cover the baking dish and marinate the ribs overnight in the refrigerator.

10. Preheat the barbecue to medium-high heat.

11. Put the ribs on the barbecue and grill them, turning, until they are browned, sizzling, and lightly caramelized, about 10 minutes.

12. Serve.

CILANTRO PORK CHOPS

PALEO-FRIENDLY GLUTEN-FREE

SERVES 4 • PREP TIME: 15 MINUTES PLUS MARINATING TIME • COOK TIME: 8 MINUTES

Marinating meat is often thought to produce a tender, flavor-packed protein, but depending on what is in the marinade, you might not get the result you want in the end. Acidic marinades, like the lime one used in this recipe, cannot be left on the pork for longer than about 30 minutes or the meat will toughen. If you need to leave the pork in the marinade longer, add a couple tablespoons of oil to cut the acidic ratio.

---

1 pound boneless center-cut pork chops, pounded to ¼-inch thickness

Sea salt

¼ cup finely chopped fresh cilantro

Juice of 2 limes

2 teaspoons minced garlic

¼ cup coconut oil

Lime wedges for garnish

1. Season the pork with salt and put in a large bowl.
2. Add the cilantro, lime juice, and garlic to the pork and use your hands to massage the marinade ingredients into the meat.
3. Set the meat aside for 30 minutes at room temperature.
4. Set a large skillet over medium-high heat and melt the coconut oil.
5. Add the pork and fry until just cooked through and still juicy, turning once, about 4 minutes per side.
6. Serve with lime wedges.

COCONUT-BANANA PORK TENDERLOIN

PALEO-FRIENDLY GLUTEN-FREE

SERVES 4 • PREP TIME: 10 MINUTES • COOK TIME: 25 MINUTES

Banana adds an exotic taste to the pork in this dish even though it is a very common fruit found in most kitchens. Although quite sweet, bananas are very versatile and can be equally delicious in savory dishes. Sautéing the banana breaks it down so that the entire sauce is infused with its tropical flavor.

---

3 tablespoons coconut oil, divided

1½ pounds boneless pork chops

1 banana, sliced thinly

1 tablespoon grated fresh ginger

1 teaspoon minced garlic

1 cup canned coconut milk

Juice of 1 lime

½ cup shredded unsweetened coconut

1. Set a large skillet over medium heat and add 2 tablespoons of oil.

2. Brown the pork on both sides, for 10 minutes total.

3. Move the pork to the side of the skillet and add the remaining oil.

4. Sauté the banana until golden, about 1 minute.

5. Stir in the ginger and garlic, and sauté for 1 minute.

6. Stir in the coconut milk and move the pork to the center of the pan.

7. Cover the skillet and simmer for 10 minutes until the meat is cooked through and tender.

8. Stir in the lime juice and serve topped with coconut.

TIP Pork is the other "white meat" with a similar nutrition profile to chicken as well as only 1 gram of fat per portion. Pork is higher in protein and has fewer calories than chicken, which makes it a wonderful choice to enjoy in your diet often.

COCONUT PORK STIR-FRY

PALEO-FRIENDLY GLUTEN-FREE

SERVES 4 • PREP TIME: 30 MINUTES • COOK TIME: 20 MINUTES

Stir-frying is a quick and healthful cooking technique that is easy to master. The best stir-frys take into account that different proteins and vegetables need different times in the skillet or wok so that they stay tender-crisp. There is not a great deal of sauce in this dish, so if you like more, double the sauce components and add a teaspoon of cornstarch to thicken the extra amount quickly.

¾ cup canned coconut milk

2 tablespoons coconut aminos

1 tablespoon honey

1 teaspoon grated fresh ginger

2 tablespoons coconut oil, divided

1 (1-pound) pork tenderloin, trimmed and cut into 1-inch cubes

1 cup broccoli florets

1 celery stalk, sliced thinly

1 carrot, peeled and cut into thin disks

½ cup sliced mushrooms

1 red bell pepper, cut into thin strips

½ cup snow peas

½ cup shredded coconut

1. In a small bowl, whisk together the coconut milk, coconut aminos, honey, and ginger. Set aside.

2. Set a large skillet over medium-high heat. Add 1 tablespoon coconut oil and heat.

3. Add the pork to the skillet and sauté until it is browned and just cooked through, about 10 minutes. Remove the pork to a plate with a slotted spoon and set aside.

4. Add the remaining coconut oil, broccoli, celery, carrot, and mushrooms to the skillet.

5. Stir-fry, tossing constantly for 5 minutes.

6. Add the red bell pepper and snow peas. Stir-fry for 3 minutes, or until the vegetables are tender-crisp.

7. Add the sauce and pork back to the skillet with any accumulated juice on the plate.

8. Toss to coat the vegetables and pork and stir-fry for 2 minutes.

9. Remove from the heat and serve topped with shredded coconut.

LAMB & LENTIL STEW

GLUTEN-FREE

SERVES 4 • PREP TIME: 20 MINUTES • COOK TIME: 40 MINUTES

Finding good-quality ground lamb can be difficult in your local supermarket because the products found in those stores are often very fatty. Try to find a butcher who can provide good-quality pasture-raised lamb, or invest in a meat grinder and grind it yourself if you use a great deal of ground meat. You can use chunks of lamb shoulder for this dish, but you will have to increase the cooking time by about 1 hour to produce tender meat.

---

2 tablespoons coconut oil

1 pound ground lamb

1 sweet onion, peeled and chopped

2 teaspoons minced fresh garlic

½ jalapeño pepper, minced

1 teaspoon grated fresh ginger

2 tablespoons tomato paste

1 teaspoon ground cumin

½ teaspoon ground cinnamon

½ teaspoon ground allspice

2 cups chicken broth

2 cups canned coconut milk

2 carrots, peeled and diced

2 sweet potatoes, peeled and diced

2 cups cooked red lentils

¼ teaspoon sea salt

2 tablespoons chopped fresh cilantro, for garnish

1. Set a large saucepan over medium-high heat and add the oil.

2. Add the ground lamb and sauté until the meat is browned, about 5 minutes.

3. Stir in the onion, garlic, jalapeño, and ginger and sauté until the vegetables are softened, about 4 minutes.

4. Stir in the tomato paste, cumin, cinnamon, and allspice until mixed.

5. Add the chicken broth, coconut milk, carrots, sweet potatoes, and lentils.

6. Bring the stew to a boil and then reduce the heat and simmer until the vegetables are tender, about 25 minutes. Stir in the salt.

7. Serve topped with cilantro.

ROSEMARY-GARLIC LAMB CHOPS

PALEO-FRIENDLY GLUTEN-FREE

SERVES 4 • PREP TIME: 10 MINUTES PLUS MARINATING TIME • COOK TIME: 15 MINUTES

Tender medium-rare lamb is a staple dish in most fine-dining restaurants because it is exceptionally tender and melds well with many herbs and seasonings. Rosemary is a classic lamb accompaniment. Rosemary comes from an evergreen shrub and has many health benefits. This pungent herb can help improve digestion, increase circulation, and boost the immune system. Try to use fresh rosemary instead of dried whenever possible because the taste is superior.

2 racks of lamb, cut into individual chops

¼ teaspoon sea salt

6 tablespoons melted coconut oil, divided

2 tablespoons chopped fresh rosemary

1 teaspoon minced garlic

1. Pat the chops dry with paper towels. Season the lamb chops with salt and place them in a single layer in a container.

2. In a small bowl, whisk together 4 tablespoons of the coconut oil, the rosemary, and the garlic until well combined.

3. Spoon the marinade over the lamb and marinate in the refrigerator, covered, for 5 hours, turning once.

4. Set a large skillet over medium-high heat, and add the remaining 2 tablespoons coconut oil.

5. Sear half the lamb chops for 2 to 3 minutes per side until they reach your desired doneness.

6. Repeat with remaining chops.

7. Let the chops rest for 5 minutes before serving.

TIP For the best results, you should use frenched lamb racks for this recipe. This means that the fat and meat is trimmed off the bones; otherwise, this task can take about 30 minutes—if you are experienced. You can also ask your butcher to do it for you or buy frenched racks for a slightly higher price.

GARAM MASALA LAMB

PALEO-FRIENDLY GLUTEN-FREE

SERVES 4 • PREP TIME: 20 MINUTES • COOK TIME: 1 HOUR 45 MINUTES

Garam masala is not curry, despite what many people think when they see it on an ingredients list. The flavor is quite different. You can make your own garam masala with a combination of spices you probably already have in your kitchen. The quantities of each spice will depend on your own taste, and the finished product will be warm and flavorful, which is logical because garam masala *means "warming spice mix." The most commonly used spices in this blend are nutmeg, fennel seed, cardamom, cinnamon, bay leaf, cumin, coriander, black pepper, and chili powder.*

---

2 tablespoons coconut oil, divided

1 pound lamb shoulder, trimmed and cut into ½-inch chunks

1 sweet onion, diced

2 celery stalks, diced

½ red chile, minced

1 tablespoon minced garlic

1½ tablespoons garam masala powder

1½ cups canned coconut milk

1 cup diced tomatoes

Juice of 1 lime

Sea salt

¼ cup parsley for garnish

1. Set a large saucepan over medium-high heat and add 1 tablespoon of the coconut oil.

2. Add the lamb and sauté until lightly browned, about 5 minutes. Remove the lamb with a slotted spoon to a plate and set aside.

3. Add the remaining oil to the saucepan and sauté the onion, celery, chile, and garlic until the vegetables are softened, about 5 minutes.

4. Add the garam masala powder and sauté for 1 additional minute.

5. Add the lamb back to the saucepan and stir in the coconut milk and diced tomatoes.

6. Bring the mixture to a boil and then reduce the heat to low so that it simmers.

7. Simmer the lamb mixture, covered, until the meat is very tender, about 1 hour 20 minutes. Stir several times while it cooks.

8. Stir in the lime juice and season with salt.

9. Serve over rice or couscous, topped with the parsley.

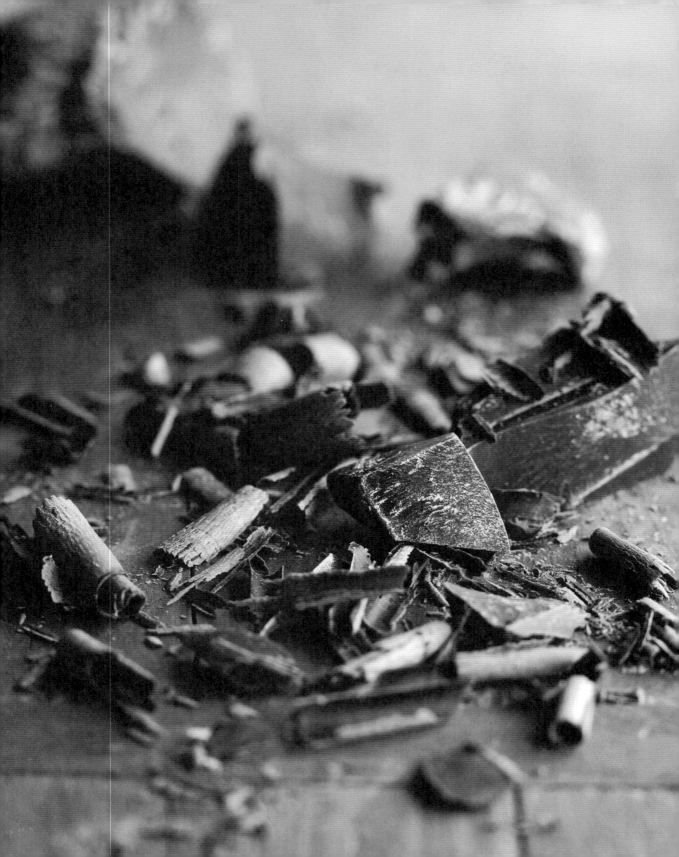

Chapter Thirteen

DESSERTS

LUSCIOUS CHOCOLATE PUDDING

VEGAN GLUTEN-FREE

SERVES 6 • PREP TIME: 5 MINUTES PLUS CHILLING TIME • COOK TIME: 5 MINUTES

Chocolate pudding is an ideal ending to a simple family meal or a rich snack before bed. This recipe has a serious chocolate flavor that could be made stronger with the addition of shaved dark chocolate as a topping. If you double the recipe, it could be used as a delectable pie filling.

---

1 (15-ounce) can coconut milk

3 cups almond milk

¾ cup cocoa powder

½ cup sugar

½ cup arrowroot flour

1 tablespoon pure vanilla extract

Pinch sea salt

¼ cup shredded coconut

1. Set a medium saucepan over medium heat and pour in the coconut milk and almond milk.

2. In a small bowl whisk together the cocoa powder, sugar, and arrowroot flour, smoothing out any lumps.

3. Whisk the cocoa mixture into the milk mixture until well blended.

4. Bring the pudding to a boil, whisking occasionally, and then whisk the mixture constantly while it boils and thickens, about 2 minutes.

5. Remove from the heat and whisk in the vanilla and salt.

6. Pour the pudding into a bowl and cover with plastic wrap so the wrap presses to the top of the pudding.

7. Chill in the refrigerator until completely cooled, for 3 hours.

8. Serve topped with shredded coconut.

LIGHT COCONUT MOUSSE

GLUTEN-FREE

SERVES 4 • PREP TIME: 15 MINUTES PLUS CHILLING TIME • COOK TIME: 8 MINUTES

The texture of mousse is a joy on the tongue, and this recipe creates a delicate, lightly flavored dessert that can be enjoyed on a warm summer evening after a satisfying meal. You can increase the coconut taste with a teaspoon of coconut extract and toasted coconut garnish, but do not add too much or you will lose the heavenly texture.

½ cup canned coconut milk

3 egg yolks

½ cup granulated sugar

1 teaspoon gelatin

¾ cup heavy (whipping) cream

1. Set a small saucepan on medium heat and add the coconut milk. Heat the milk until it is just boiling and remove from the stove.

2. In a bowl, whisk together the yolks and sugar until blended.

3. Whisk the coconut milk into the yolks and return the mixture to the saucepan.

4. Put the saucepan over medium heat and whisk until the mixture thickens, about 3 minutes.

5. Remove from the heat and whisk in the gelatin.

6. Transfer the mixture to a medium bowl and put it in the refrigerator to cool completely, about 1 hour.

7. Pour the whipping cream into a medium bowl, and with an electric hand beater set on medium speed, whip the cream until it is thickened, about 3 minutes.

8. When the coconut mixture is cool, fold in the whipped cream until the mousse is fluffy and well combined.

9. Serve.

COCONUT BREAD PUDDING

SERVES 10 • PREP TIME: 15 MINUTES PLUS SOAKING TIME • COOK TIME: 1 HOUR

Bread pudding started as a tasty way to use up stale bread in the 11th century and has evolved into a spectacular dessert featured in the finest restaurants in the world. There are countless variations of this recipe because the basic recipe is very forgiving. The coconut version of bread pudding found here would taste sublime with a handful of chocolate chips or dried cranberries. Experiment with different ingredients until you hit on a favorite combination.

Coconut oil for greasing the pan

1 (15-ounce) can coconut milk

4 large eggs

½ cup plus 4 tablespoons sugar, divided

2 teaspoons pure vanilla extract

14 cups cubed French bread with crust (12 ounces)

½ cup shredded unsweetened coconut

½ cup chopped pecans

1. Preheat the oven to 350°F.

2. Grease a 13-by-9-by-3-inch glass baking dish with coconut oil.

3. In a large bowl, whisk together the coconut milk, eggs, ½ cup of the sugar, and the vanilla.

4. Add the bread, coconut, and pecans to the coconut milk mixture and stir so that the bread is soaked. Let the mixture sit for 30 minutes and then transfer it to the baking dish.

5. Bake the pudding until the edges are golden and the custard is set in the center, about 1 hour. Sprinkle the remaining 4 tablespoons of sugar on top.

6. Cool the pudding slightly and serve.

COCONUT ICE MILK

PALEO-FRIENDLY GLUTEN-FREE

SERVES 4 • PREP TIME: 15 MINUTES PLUS CHILLING TIME • COOK TIME: 0 MINUTES

Intense coconut flavor is the result of three kinds of coconut in this recipe. If you want a delightful variation, add a cup of mini chocolate chips to create an ice cream that tastes like a popular candy bar. Full-fat coconut milk will create the creamiest dessert, but if you are counting calories, light coconut milk tastes lovely, too. The coconut extract is an important component in this recipe, so try to obtain pure extract rather than imitation for better quality.

4 cups canned coconut milk

½ cup honey

1 teaspoon coconut extract

2 cups shredded unsweetened coconut

1. In a medium bowl, whisk together the coconut milk, honey, and coconut extract until well blended.

2. Add the coconut and stir to combine.

3. Transfer the coconut mixture to an ice cream maker and freeze according to the manufacturer's directions.

COCONUT-MANGO ICE POPS

PALEO-FRIENDLY GLUTEN-FREE

SERVES 8 • PREP TIME: 15 MINUTES PLUS FREEZING TIME • COOK TIME: 0 MINUTES

Sitting in the warm summer sun while licking a dripping ice pop is an enjoyable childhood experience for most, and these homemade ice pops elevate that simple pleasure into a sophisticated treat. If you want to create a spectacular presentation, omit the mango from the blender at first and create a pale coconut liquid. Use half of the coconut liquid to fill the ice pop mold halfway, then add the mango to the remaining coconut liquid in the blender, blend until smooth, and fill the pop molds the rest of the way with this brighter mixture.

---

1 (15-ounce) can coconut milk

1 mango, peeled, pitted, and chopped

¼ cup shredded coconut

¼ cup honey

Zest and juice of 1 lime

1. Put the coconut milk, mango, coconut, honey, and lime zest and juice in a blender and blend until smooth.

2. Pour the mixture into ice pop molds and freeze.

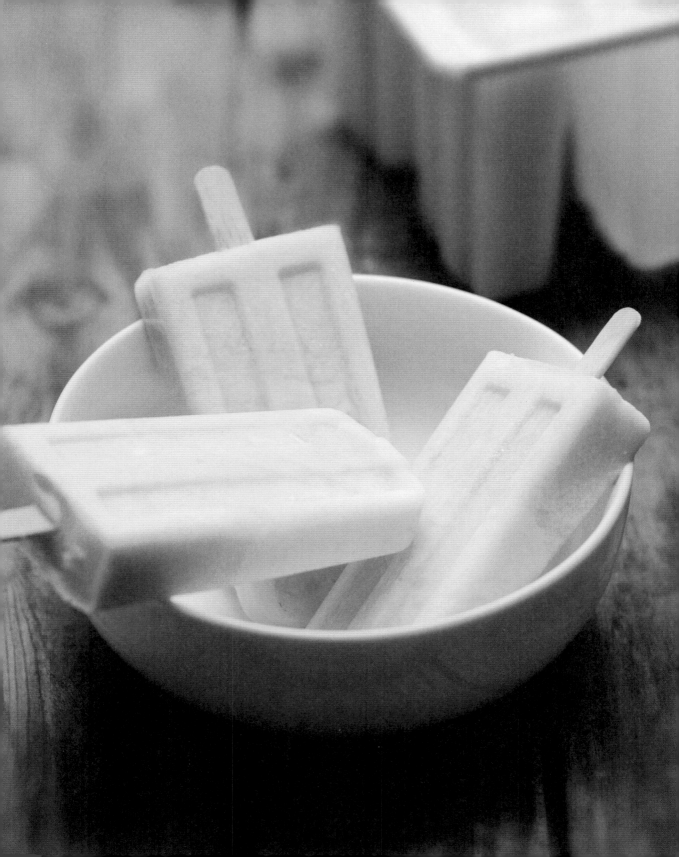

FRENCH VANILLA ICE CREAM

PALEO-FRIENDLY VEGAN GLUTEN-FREE

MAKES 6 CUPS • PREP TIME: 15 MINUTES PLUS CHILLING TIME • COOK TIME: 0 MINUTES

You will need an ice cream maker to get the creamy texture of traditional ice cream. If you do not have this piece of equipment, you can freeze the mixture in a deep metal baking dish and keep stirring it as it solidifies. The texture will not be as smooth, but the taste will still be incredible.

---

3 cups chopped fresh coconut

2 cups canned coconut milk

1 cup almond milk

1 cup maple syrup

¼ cup coconut oil

1 tablespoon pure vanilla extract

1. Put the coconut, coconut milk, almond milk, maple syrup, coconut oil, and vanilla in a blender and blend until very smooth and creamy.

2. Transfer the vanilla mixture to an ice cream maker and freeze according to the manufacturer's directions.

COCONUT RICE PUDDING

VEGAN GLUTEN-FREE

SERVES 4 • PREP TIME: 15 MINUTES • COOK TIME: 30 MINUTES

Rice pudding is a staple in many cultures because it is a simple comforting food that can fill you up as a whole meal or end a spectacular dinner on the right note as a dessert. Rice will soak up any liquid, and coconut milk creates a tender creamy porridge instead of individual grains. If you want to intensify the vanilla flavor in this dessert, infuse the milk with a scraped vanilla bean pod first. This will also add interesting black flecks to the pudding from the vanilla seeds.

---

2 cups canned light coconut milk, divided

1 cup almond milk

1¼ cups basmati rice

½ cup granulated sugar

Pinch sea salt

1 teaspoon pure vanilla extract

½ cup shredded unsweetened coconut

1. Set a medium saucepan over medium-heat heat and add 1½ cups coconut milk, almond milk, rice, sugar, salt, and vanilla.

2. Bring the rice mixture to a boil and then reduce the heat to low and simmer.

3. Simmer until the rice is tender, stirring frequently, about 25 minutes.

4. Remove the pudding from the heat and stir in the remaining coconut milk and coconut.

5. Serve warm.

ELEGANT COCONUT CRÈME BRÛLÉE

GLUTEN-FREE

SERVES 4 • PREP TIME: 15 MINUTES • COOK TIME: 1 HOUR

Crème brûlée is French for "burnt cream," which refers to the caramelized sugar topping on this creamy pudding. Many home cooks do not have access to the broiler that is used for caramelizing sugar or the butane torches that are common in professional kitchens. To make the preparation easier, this recipe has a toasted coconut topping instead of crunchy sugar. Use sweetened coconut when toasting it so you get that bittersweet caramel taste from the added sugar.

1 (15-ounce) can coconut milk

½ cup granulated sugar

1 tablespoon arrowroot flour

8 egg yolks

4 teaspoons toasted coconut

1. Preheat the oven to 300°F.

2. Place 4 (6-ounce) ramekins in a baking dish and set aside.

3. Set a small saucepan on medium heat. Pour in the coconut milk and heat until it is just below boiling, and remove from the stove.

4. In a medium bowl, stir together the sugar and arrowroot flour and then whisk in the egg yolks.

5. Whisk the coconut milk into the yolk mixture until blended.

6. Pour the brûlée mix through a fine sieve into a large measuring cup.

7. Pour the mix equally into the ramekins and pour water into the baking dish so that the water comes up an inch on the sides of the ramekins. Take care not to get any water into the ramekins.

8. Bake the crème brûlée until the puddings are firm but the centers still move a little when the pan is shaken gently, about 50 minutes.

9. Remove the ramekins from the baking sheet and chill the crème brûlée completely before serving. Top with toasted coconut.

TIP For a traditional crème brûlée, sprinkle the tops of each pudding with a thin coating of granulated sugar and use a handheld torch to caramelize the sugar into a crunchy golden crust.

LEMON & COCONUT TRUFFLES

PALEO-FRIENDLY GLUTEN-FREE

MAKES 16 TRUFFLES • PREP TIME: 30 MINUTES • COOK TIME: 0 MINUTES

Puréed coconut and cashews form the base for these perfectly balanced truffles. They are sweet and tart with a luscious texture. You can use two limes instead of lemon to create Key lime truffles, or a combination of both citrus fruits. You will need to mince the zest very well so that there are no long strings in the truffles.

---

3 cups shredded unsweetened coconut, divided

½ cup cashews

¼ cup honey

2 tablespoons coconut oil

Zest of 1 lemon, finely minced

Juice of 1 lemon

1. Put 2 cups of coconut and the cashews in a food processor and blend until the mixture starts to look like a paste, about 5 minutes.

2. Add the honey, coconut oil, lemon zest, and lemon juice to the processor and blend until the mixture forms a ball, about 2 minutes.

3. Roll the coconut mixture into 16 balls and roll the balls generously in the remaining coconut.

4. Store the truffles in a sealed container in the refrigerator for up to 1 week.

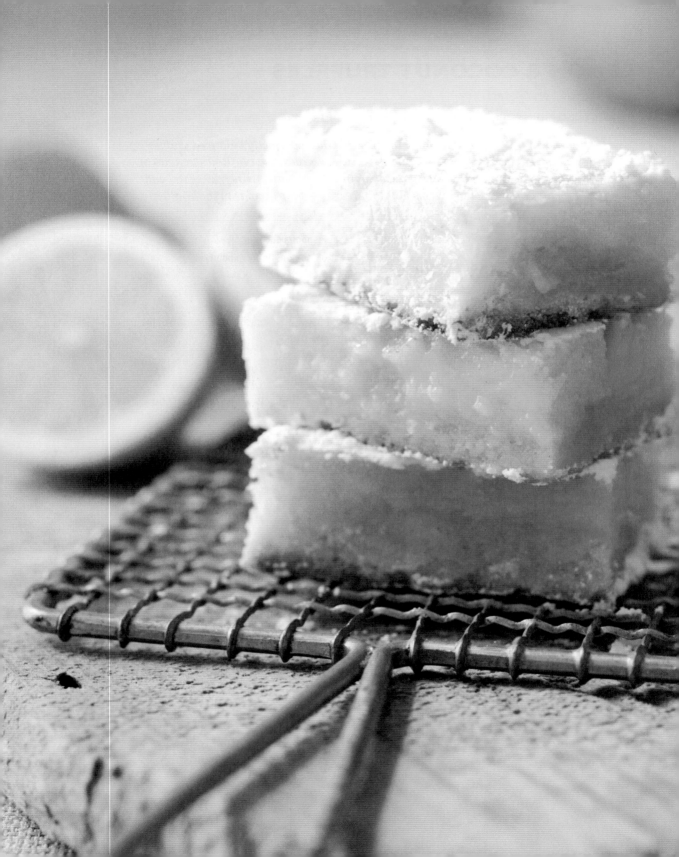

LUSCIOUS LEMON BARS

GLUTEN-FREE

MAKES 16 BARS • PREP TIME: 15 MINUTES PLUS CHILLING TIME • COOK TIME: 0 MINUTES

This pretty, no-bake bar will remind you of lemon meringue pie because of the assertive citrus flavor. The crust is held together by sweet dates, and tastes like a chewy granola bar. Dates provide energy and are often the snack of choice for athletes. Dates are high in iron, fiber, vitamin A, and many antioxidants that can boost your immunity and promote a healthy digestive system.

For the base

1 cup large-flake gluten-free oats

1 cup shredded unsweetened coconut

1 cup dates, pitted

For the lemon layer

1 can condensed milk

Juice from 3 lemons

1 cup shredded unsweetened coconut

2 tablespoons coconut oil, melted

Powdered sugar for dusting

To make the base

1. Put the oats, coconut, and dates in a food processor and pulse until the mixture sticks together.

2. Press the base mixture into the bottom of an 8-by-8-inch baking pan and put it in the refrigerator just until chilled.

To make the lemon layer

1. In a medium bowl, whisk together the condensed milk, lemon juice, coconut, and coconut oil until well blended.

2. Spread the lemon layer onto the chilled base and put the pan back in the refrigerator.

3. Chill for at least 12 hours.

4. Dust with powdered sugar and cut into squares. Store them in the refrigerator for up to 1 week.

TIP These bars can be gluten-free if you buy oats that are labeled gluten-free. Oats themselves do not contain gluten, but many products are manufactured in plants that also process other gluten-containing grains, so there is a risk of cross-contamination.

PERFECT COCONUT MACAROONS

PALEO-FRIENDLY **VEGAN** GLUTEN-FREE

MAKES 16 COOKIES • PREP TIME: 10 MINUTES PLUS CHILLING TIME • COOK TIME: 1½ HOURS

Macaroons have a long, interesting history that started without the addition of coconut—just ground almond and egg whites instead. This recipe uses both almond flour and coconut but excludes the beaten egg whites. Do not substitute sweetened coconut for unsweetened, or these cookies might be too sweet. You can drizzle some melted dark chocolate across your macaroons for a delicious variation.

1½ cups shredded unsweetened coconut

¼ cup almond flour

½ teaspoon ground cinnamon

Pinch sea salt

6 tablespoons maple syrup

3 tablespoons coconut oil, melted

1 teaspoon pure vanilla extract

1. Preheat the oven to 200°F.
2. Line a baking sheet with parchment paper. Set aside.
3. In a large bowl, stir together the coconut, almond flour, cinnamon, and salt.
4. In a small bowl, whisk together the maple syrup, coconut oil, and vanilla.
5. Add the maple mixture to the coconut mixture and stir to combine.
6. Put the batter in the refrigerator and chill until it can be scooped easily, about 15 minutes.
7. Drop the cookie batter by tablespoons onto the prepared baking sheet, about 1 inch apart.
8. Bake the cookies for about 1½ hours, or until firm and dry on the outside.
9. Cool on a rack and store in a sealed container in a cool spot for up to 1 week.

DELECTABLE CHOCOLATE FUDGE

VEGAN GLUTEN-FREE

MAKES 30 PIECES • PREP TIME: 15 MINUTES PLUS CHILLING TIME • COOK TIME: 0 MINUTES

Traditional fudge is a scrumptious treat that can be difficult to make if you do not know how to create soft ball sugar, and do not time everything perfectly. This fudge is easy to make, and you will not need a thermometer. It also turns out creamy and smooth with hardly any work. Make sure you use good-quality cocoa powder so that the chocolate flavor is deep and rich.

---

1 cup coconut oil, melted

¾ cup cocoa powder

½ cup confectioner's sugar

1 teaspoon vanilla

Pinch sea salt

1. Line a 9-by-9-inch glass baking dish with plastic wrap and set aside.

2. Pour the melted coconut oil into a food processor and sift in the cocoa and confectioner's sugar. Process the mixture until just blended.

3. Add the vanilla and salt to the food processor and process until well blended.

4. Spoon the fudge mixture into the prepared baking dish and press it down using another sheet of plastic wrap over the top.

5. Put the dish in the refrigerator and chill until the fudge is set up and firm, about 3 hours.

6. Remove the fudge from the dish and cut it into pieces.

7. Store the fudge in the refrigerator in a sealed container for up to 1 month.

DOUBLE-COCONUT CHEESECAKE

SERVES 12 • PREP TIME: 25 MINUTES PLUS CHILLING TIME • COOK TIME: 1 HOUR 10 MINUTES PLUS 50 MINUTES

Cheesecake is a sublime indulgence that is almost sinful in nature. The lush excess of this coconut-packed dessert is the perfect end to a special evening with family and friends. Make sure your coconut milk is a full-fat product to get the right texture and flavor in the filling. If you want to continue the coconut theme further, place a can of full-fat coconut milk or coconut cream in the refrigerator, and the heavy cream will rise to the top and solidify. With an electric hand beater, whip the coconut cream into a fluffy whipped topping and add toasted coconut as the final garnish.

For the crust

1 cup graham cracker crumbs

½ cup shredded unsweetened coconut

¼ cup granulated sugar

4 tablespoons butter, melted

For the cheesecake

1½ pounds cream cheese, at room temperature

1 cup granulated sugar

4 large eggs

½ cup canned coconut milk

1 tablespoon all-purpose flour

1 tablespoon pure vanilla extract

1 teaspoon coconut extract

¼ teaspoon sea salt

To make the crust

1. Preheat the oven to 350°F.

2. In a bowl, stir together the graham cracker crumbs, coconut, and sugar until well mixed.

3. Add the melted butter and stir until the mixture resembles coarse crumbs.

4. Press the graham cracker mixture into the bottom and halfway up the sides of a 9-inch springform pan.

5. Bake the crust until light golden brown, for 10 minutes.

6. Remove the crust from the oven and allow it to cool.

To make the cheesecake

1. Reduce the oven temperature to 325ºF.

2. In a medium bowl, using an electric hand beater set on medium speed, beat the cream cheese until it is very smooth, scraping down the sides and bottom of the bowl often.

3. Beat in the sugar until smooth and combined.

4. Add the eggs to the bowl one at a time, beating well and scraping down the sides of the bowl between each addition.

5. Beat in the coconut milk, flour, vanilla, coconut extract, and salt until combined.

6. Pour the cheesecake mixture into the prepared crust.

7. Put the springform pan in a large baking dish and add enough hot water until it reaches halfway up the sides of the pan.

8. Bake on the center rack of the oven until the filling is set and only slightly shakes in the center, for 50 minutes.

9. Carefully remove the baking dish from the oven and then remove the springform pan.

10. Run a knife around the outside of the cheesecake and then allow it to cool to room temperature.

11. Refrigerate the cheesecake for around 8 hours to chill completely.

12. Remove the cheesecake from the springform pan and serve.

TIP Always beat your cream cheese and eggs at room temperature, or you will not be able to get your batter silky smooth. You also need to beat out all the lumps in the cream cheese before adding any other ingredients, because it is impossible to remove lumps after the batter is thinned out.

COCONUT-VANILLA BUNDT CAKE

SERVES 12 • PREP TIME: 20 MINUTES • COOK TIME: 1 HOUR

This golden cake is an ideal choice for Sunday brunch, a baby shower, a pretty gift for a hostess, or simply as a delicious after-school snack. The tender crumbed texture and subtle vanilla flavor is just right when you want a treat that is not too filling. Try using fresh berries or a lightly sweetened coconut glaze as a topping if you want to use this humble cake as a dessert.

Coconut oil for greasing the pan

All-purpose flour for dusting the pan

½ cup butter, at room temperature

½ cup coconut oil, softened

2 cups granulated sugar

6 large eggs

1 tablespoon vanilla extract

2 cups all-purpose flour

1¼ cups almond flour

⅓ cup cornstarch

1 teaspoon baking powder

1 teaspoon sea salt

1 (15-ounce) can unsweetened coconut milk

2 cups shredded sweetened coconut

1. Preheat the oven to 350°F.

2. Grease and flour a 12-cup Bundt pan and set aside.

3. In a large bowl, cream together the butter, coconut oil, and sugar with an electric hand beater until fluffy, about 5 minutes.

4. Beat in the eggs one at a time, scraping down the sides of the bowl after each egg.

5. Beat in the vanilla.

6. In another bowl, whisk together the all-purpose flour, almond flour, cornstarch, baking powder, and salt until well mixed.

7. Stir the coconut milk and flour mixture into the butter-and-egg mixture in five increments, starting and ending with the flour mixture.

8. Stir in the shredded coconut.

9. Spoon the batter into the prepared Bundt pan and bake until a toothpick inserted into the center of the cake comes out clean, about 1 hour.

10. Cool the cake for 30 minutes in the pan, then carefully invert it onto a rack and let it cool to room temperature.

11. Serve.

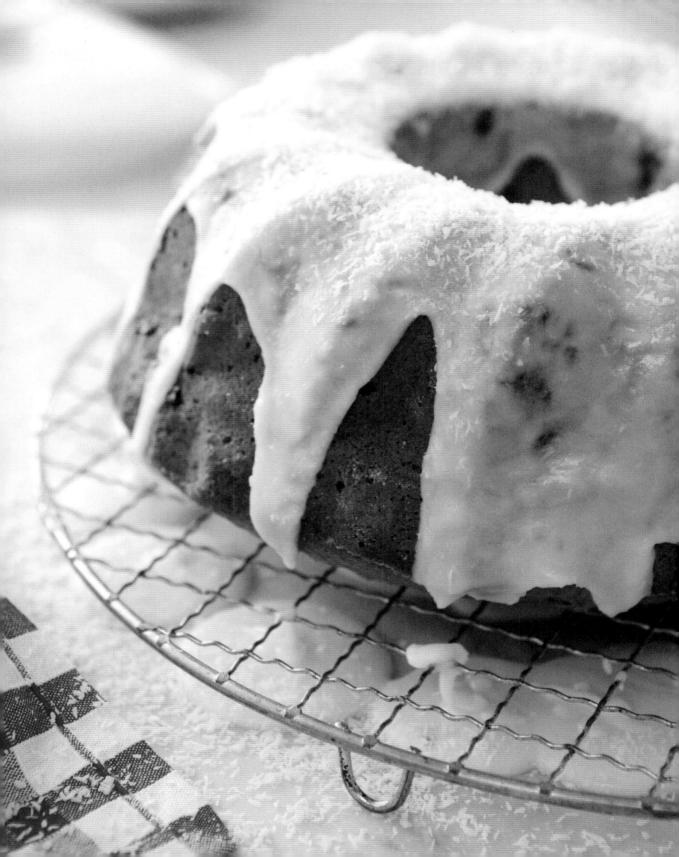

PEAR & APPLE COCONUT CRISP

VEGAN

SERVES 8 • PREP TIME: 15 MINUTES • COOK TIME: 35 MINUTES

This crisp is exceptionally high in fiber. Apples, pears, oats, coconut, and even the cinnamon add fiber to the dish. Fiber is important to general good health because it can help reduce the risk of colon cancer, regulate blood sugar, and promote a healthy digestive system. You can increase the fiber by leaving the skins on your pears after washing them thoroughly. Pear skin also contains three times more phenolic phytonutrients than the flesh of the fruit, so it is a healthful addition to the recipe.

½ cup plus 1 tablespoon melted coconut oil, divided

3 pears, peeled, cored, and cut into slices

3 apples, peeled, cored, and cut into slices

1 teaspoon ground cinnamon, divided

1 cup large-flake oats

½ cup brown sugar

½ cup chopped pecans

¼ cup all-purpose flour

¼ cup coconut flour

½ teaspoon allspice

¼ teaspoon sea salt

1. Preheat the oven to 375°F.

2. Set a medium skillet over medium heat and melt 1 tablespoon of the coconut oil.

3. Sauté the pears and apples until tender-crisp, about 4 minutes.

4. Stir in ½ teaspoon of the cinnamon and transfer the fruit to a 9-by-9-inch glass baking dish. Set aside.

5. In a large bowl, toss together the oats, sugar, pecans, all-purpose flour, coconut flour, allspice, salt, and the remaining ½ teaspoon cinnamon until well mixed.

6. Add the remaining ½ cup melted coconut oil and toss until the mixture resembles coarse crumbs.

7. Top the fruit evenly with the crumble mixture.

8. Bake the crisp until golden, about 30 minutes.

9. Serve warm.

TIP Stay away from quick or instant oats when making the crisp part of this dish, because they will not give you the right texture. Large-flake or rolled oats form a crispy topping that still breaks easily into buttery clumps, unlike quick oats, which form a more solid cookie-like top that is hard to get a fork through.

TRADITIONAL COCONUT CREAM PIE

GLUTEN-FREE

SERVES 8 • PREP TIME: 20 MINUTES PLUS COOLING TIME • COOK TIME: 10 MINUTES

Cream pies look luxurious, and coconut cream pie is the ultimate indulgence, with layers of lovely coconut-infused pastry cream and clouds of whipped cream. Take the time to toast the coconut for the topping because toasting intensifies the flavor, and the golden brown color is a beautiful contrast to the snowy whipped cream.

1 cup shredded unsweetened coconut

2 (15-ounce) cans coconut milk

½ cup arrowroot flour

1 cup granulated sugar, divided

2 teaspoons pure vanilla extract, divided

1 teaspoon coconut extract

¼ teaspoon sea salt

1 prepared deep dish crust, baked and cooled

2 cups heavy (whipping) cream

1. Preheat the oven to 350°F.

2. Line a baking sheet with parchment paper.

3. Spread the coconut on the baking sheet and toast in the oven until golden brown, about 5 minutes.

4. Remove the coconut from the oven and set aside to cool.

5. Pour the coconut milk into a medium saucepan and whisk in the arrowroot flour, ½ cup sugar, 1 teaspoon vanilla, coconut extract, and salt.

6. Put the saucepan over medium heat and bring the mixture to a boil, stirring frequently, about 4 minutes. Continue boiling the mixture for 1 minute to thicken.

7. Remove from the heat and pour the filling into the prepared crust.

8. Put the pie in the refrigerator to cool for 1 hour.

9. Pour the whipping cream into a medium bowl and, using an electric hand beater set on medium speed, whip the cream until it thickens, about 4 minutes.

10. Add the remaining ½ cup sugar and 1 teaspoon vanilla and whip until the cream is fluffy.

11. Top the cooled pie with mounds of whipped cream and top with toasted coconut.

12. Serve.

COCONUT LAYER CAKE WITH FLUFFY TOASTED-COCONUT FROSTING

SERVES 12 • PREP TIME: 20 MINUTES • COOK TIME: 30 MINUTES

You will have to bake this cake again and again for family events because the cake is tender, the frosting buttery, and the double-coconut flavor superb. You can bake this as a sheet cake if you do not need a three-layer creation, but you will need to increase the baking time by 10 minutes. This cake can be made ahead and frozen for up to 2 weeks if you want to save time closer to your event.

For coconut cake
Coconut oil for greasing the pans
All-purpose flour for dusting the pans
1½ cups butter, at room temperature
3 cups granulated sugar
6 large eggs
1 teaspoon pure coconut extract
4 cups sifted all-purpose flour
1 teaspoon baking powder
1½ teaspoons baking soda

Pinch sea salt
¼ teaspoon ground nutmeg
1½ cups canned coconut milk

For coconut frosting
16 ounces cream cheese, at room temperature
1 cup butter, at room temperature
3 to 4 cups confectioner's sugar
2 teaspoons fresh lime juice
1 teaspoon pure vanilla extract
3 cups shredded coconut, toasted lightly

To make the coconut cake

1. Preheat the oven to 350ºF.

2. Prepare three (9-inch) cake pans by greasing them lightly and dusting them with flour; set aside.

3. In a large bowl, using an electric hand beater, cream together the butter and sugar until the mixture is very light and fluffy, approximately 5 to 7 minutes.

4. Add the eggs one at a time, beating well after each addition. Scrape down the sides of the bowl after all the eggs have been added to the batter. Beat in the coconut extract.

5. In a medium bowl, sift together the all-purpose flour, baking powder, baking soda, salt, and nutmeg.

6. Beat the coconut milk and dry ingredients into a creamed mixture, alternating in batches starting and ending with the dry ingredients. Beat this creamed mixture into the egg batter. Scrape down the sides of the bowl to ensure that everything is well incorporated.

7. Divide the batter evenly among the three prepared pans and bake on the top rack of the preheated oven for 28 to 30 minutes, or until a toothpick inserted into the center of the cakes comes out clean.

8. Remove the cakes from the oven and allow them to cool for at least 15 minutes in their pans. Then carefully invert them onto racks to finish cooling. Allow the cakes to cool completely before frosting them.

To make the coconut frosting

1. In a large bowl using an electric hand beater, beat together the cream cheese and butter until the mixture is completely smooth and fluffy. Add the confectioner's sugar a little at a time until the frosting reaches your desired level of sweetness. Beat in the lime juice and vanilla extract.

2. Fill the cooled cake layers with the frosting and then frost the filled, stacked cake with swirls and texture. Coat the sides and top with the toasted coconut.

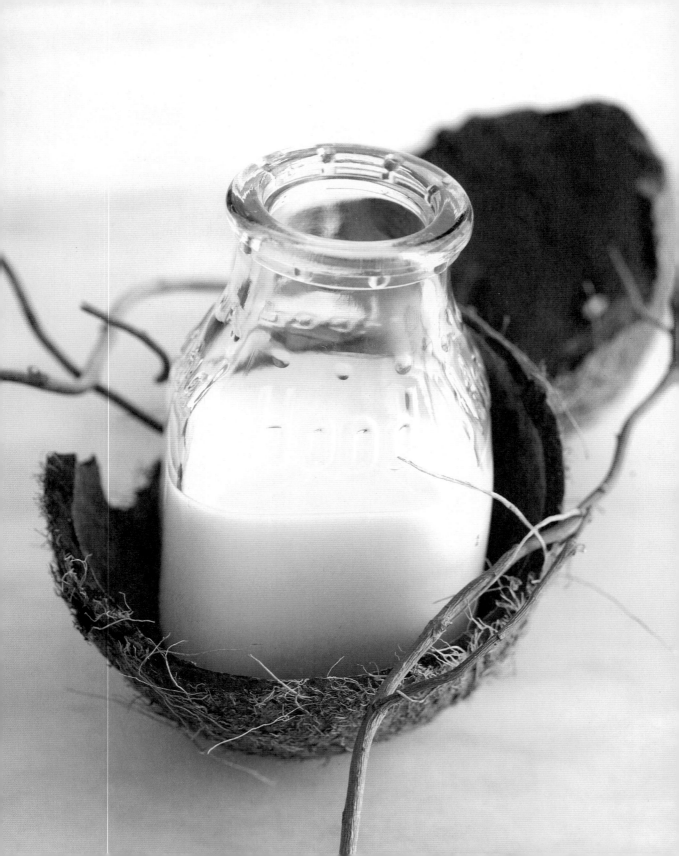

RESOURCES

Books

Blanco, Maria, and James Pendleton. *The Complete Idiot's Guide to the Coconut Oil Diet.* Alpha Books, 2013.

Fife, Bruce. *Coconut Cures: Preventing and Treating Common Health Problems with Coconut.* Picadilly Books, 2005.

Fife, Bruce. *The Coconut Oil Miracle.* Penguin, 2013.

Fife, Bruce. *Oil Pulling Therapy: Detoxifying and Healing the Body Through Oral Cleansing.* Picadilly Books, 2008.

Gursche, Siegfried. *Coconut Oil: The Healthiest Oil on Earth.* Book Publishing Co., 2008.

Holzapfel, Cynthia. *Coconut Oil for Health and Beauty.* Book Publishing Co., 2003.

Moro, Halina. *Coconut Oil: 100 Most Crucial Questions Answered.* Amazon Digital Services, 2013.

Nyland, Elizabeth. *Cooking with Coconut Oil: Gluten-Free, Grain-Free Recipes for Good Living.* Countryman Press, 2014.

Rockridge Press. *Cooking with Coconut Oil: Your Coconut Oil Miracle Guide: Health Cures, Beauty, Weight Loss, and Delicious Recipes.* Rockridge Press, 2013.

Sterling, Samatha. *Cooking with Coconut Oil: 50 Coconut Oil Recipes Promoting Health, Wellness, & Beauty. Vol. 1.* CreateSpace, 2014.

Stone, Linda. *Coconut Oil: The Ultimate Guide to Coconut Oil: The Benefits, Cures, Uses and Remedies of Coconut Oil.* Amazon Digital Services, 2014.

Wiggins, Darrin. *50 Weight Loss Shakes: Lose Weight Naturally with Coconut Oil and Coconut Milk Smoothies.* CreateSpace, 2015.

Wright, Jamie. *The Coconut Oil Handbook: How to Lose Weight, Improve Cholesterol, Alleviate Allergies, Renew Your Skin, and Get Healthier with Coconut Oil.* CreateSpace, 2013.

Websites

Coconut Research Center:
www.coconutresearchcenter.org/index.htm

Coconut Oil:
coconutoil.com

Coconut Oil Cures:
www.earthclinic.com/remedies/coconut_oil.html

Coconut Oil Cooking:
coconutoilcooking.com

Coconut Oil Diet:
www.coconutdiet.com

Amazing Beauty Tips for Coconut:
www.prevention.com/beauty/natural-beauty/coconut-oil-cures-your-skin-and-hair

101 Uses for Coconut Oil:
wellnessmama.com/5734/101-uses-for-coconut-oil/

REFERENCES

Agero, A.L., and V.M. Verallo-Rowell. "A Randomized Double-Blind Controlled Trial Comparing Virgin Coconut Oil with Mineral Oil as a Moisturizer for Mild to Moderate Xerosis." *Dermatitis* 15, no. 3: (September 2004): 109–16.

Altshul, Sara. "Sweet Scent of Sleep." *Prevention* 58, no. 7: (July 2006): 94

Asokan, S., J. Rathan, M.S. Muthu, P.V. Rathna, P. Emmadi, Raghuraman, and Chamundeswari. "Effect of Oil Pulling on *Streptococcus Mutans* Count in Plaque and Saliva Using Dentocult SM Strip Mutans Test: A Randomized, Controlled, Triple-Blind Study." *Journal of the Indian Society of Periodontics and Preventive Dentistry* 26, no. 1: (March 2008): 12–17. doi:10.4103/0970-4388.40315.

Assunção, M.L., H.S. Ferreira, A.F. dos Santos, C.R. Cabral Jr., and T.M. Florêncio. "Effects of Dietary Coconut Oil on the Biochemical and Anthropometric Profiles of Women Presenting Abdominal Obesity." *Lipids* 44, no. 7: (July 2009): 593–601. doi:10.1007/s11745-009-3306-6.

Baba N., E.F. Bracco, and S.A. Hashim. "Enhanced Thermogenesis and Diminished Deposition of Fat in Response to Overfeeding with Diet Containing Medium Chain Triglyceride." *American Journal of Clinical Nutrition* 35, no. 4: (April 1982): 678–82.

Batovska, D.I., I.T. Todorova, I.V. Tsvetkova, and H.M. Najdenski. "Antibacterial Study of the Medium Chain Fatty Acids and Their 1-Monoglycerides: Individual Effects and Synergistic Relationships." *Polish Journal of Microbiology* 58, no. 1 (2009): 43–7.

Baudouin, L., B. F. Gunn, and K. M. Olsen. "The Presence of Coconut in Southern Panama in Pre-Columbian Times: Clearing Up the Confusion." *Annals of Botany* 113 (2014): 1–5. doi:10.1093/aob/mct244.

Bio. "James Cook." Accessed Feb 29, 2015. www.biography.com/people/james-cook-21210409.

Campbell-Falck, D., T. Thomas, T.M. Falck, N. Tutuo, and K. Clem. "The Intravenous Use of Coconut Water." *American Journal of Emergency Medicine* 18, no. 1 (January 2000): 108–11.

Cardiff University. "A Wise Man's Treatment for Arthritis: Frankincense?" ScienceDaily, August 4, 2011. Accessed February 17, 2015. www.sciencedaily.com/releases/2011/06/110621121316.htm.

Clampitt, Cynthia. "A Lovely Bunch of Coconuts." *Worlds Fare.* Accessed February 18, 2015. worldsfare.wordpress.com/2008/04/14/a-lovely-bunch-of-coconuts.

Clegg, M.E., M. Golsorkhi, and C.J. Henry. "Combined Medium-Chain Triglyceride and Chili Feeding Increases Diet-Induced Thermogenesis in Normal-Weight Humans." *European Journal of Nutrition* 52, no. 6 (September 2013): 1579–85. doi:10.1007/s00394-012-0463-9.

Conlon, L.E., R.D. King, N.E. Moran, and J.W. Erdman Jr. "Coconut Oil Enhances Tomato Carotenoid Tissue Accumulation Compared to Safflower Oil in the Mongolian Gerbil (*Meriones unguiculatus*)." *Journal of Agriculture and Food Chemistry* 29, no. 60 (34) (August 2012): 8386–94. doi:10.1021/jf301902k.

Eing, M.G. "Health and Nutritional Benefits from Coconut Oil: An Important Functional Food for the 21st Century." *The Weston A. Price Foundation*. Accessed February 19, 2015. www.westonaprice.org/health-topics/a-new-look-at-coconut-oil/.

Enig, M.G. *Know Your Fats: The Complete Primer for Understanding the Nutrition of Fats, Oils, and Cholesterol*. Bethesda, MD: Bethesda Press, 2000.

Fife, Bruce. *The Coconut Oil Miracle*. 5th Ed. New York, NY: Avery, 2013

Hierholzer, J.C., and J.J. Kabara. "In Vitro Effects on Monolaurin Compounds on Enveloped RNA and DNA Viruses." *Journal of Food Safety* 4: (1982): 1–12. doi:10.1111/j.1745-4565.1982.tb00429.

Hornell, James. "Was There Pre-Columbian Contact Between the Peoples of Oceania and South America?" *The Journal of Polynesian Society* 54, no.4 (1945): 167–191.

Intahphuak, S., P. Khonsung, and A. Panthong. "Anti-Inflammatory, Analgesic, and Antipyretic Activities of Virgin Coconut Oil." *Pharmaceutical Biology* 48, no. 2 (February 2010): 151–57 doi:10.3109/13880200903062614.

Jacob, Aglaée. "Coconut Oil — Learn More About This Superfood That Contains Healthful Saturated Fats." *Today's Dietitian* 15, no. 10: 56.

Kabara, J.J. "Antimicrobial Agents Derived from Fatty Acids." *Journal of the American Oil Chemists' Society* 61 (1984): 397–403. doi:10.1007/BF02678802.

Kasai, M., N. Nosaka, H. Maki, Y. Suzuki, H. Takeuchi, T. Aoyama, A. Ohra, et al. "Comparison of Diet-Induced Thermogenesis of Foods Containing Medium- Versus Long-Chain Triacylglycerols." *Journal of Nutritional Science* 48, no. 6 (December 2002): 536–40.

Kaunitz, H. "Nutritional Properties of Coconut Oil." *Journal of the American Oil Chemists' Society* 47 (1970): 462A–66A.

Kochikuzhyil, B.M., K. Devi, and S.R. Fattepur. "Effect of Saturated Fatty Acid-Rich Dietary Vegetable Oils on Lipid Profile, Antioxidant Enzymes and Glucose Tolerance in Diabetic Rats." *Indian Journal of Pharmacology* 42, no. 3 (June 2010): 142–45. doi:10.4103/0253-7613.66835.

Labarthe, F., R. Gélinas, and C. Des Rosiers. "Medium-Chain Fatty Acids as Metabolic Therapy in Cardiac Disease." *Cardiovascular Drugs Therapy* 22, no. 2 (April 2008): 97–106. doi:10.1007/s10557-008-6084-0.

Liu, Y.M., and H.S. Wang. "Medium-Chain Triglyceride Ketogenic Diet, an Effective Treatment for Drug-Resistant Epilepsy and a Comparison with Other Ketogenic Diets." *Biomedical Journal* 36, no.1 (January 2013): 9–15. doi:10.4103/2319-4170.107154.

Marina, A.M., Y.B. Man, S.A. Nazimah, and I. Amin. "Antioxidant Capacity and Phenolic Acids of Virgin Coconut Oil." *International Journal of Food Science and Nutrition* 60, no. 2 (2209): 114–23. doi:10.1080/09637480802549127.

Mensink, R.O., P.L. Zock, A.D. Kester, and M.B. Katan. "Effects of Dietary Fatty Acids and Carbohydrates on the Ratio of Serum Total to HDL Cholesterol and on Serum Lipids and Apolipoproteins: A Meta-analysis of 60 Controlled Trials." *American Journal of Clinical Nutrition* 77, no. 5 (May 2003): 1146–55.

Mintel. "Launches of Coconut Water Quadruple over the Past Five Years." *Italian Food and Beverage Technology*, September 2013. issuu.com/chied/docs/ibt13-02web.

Nakatsuji, T., M.C. Kao, J.Y. Fang, C.C. Zouboulis, L. Zhang, R.L. Gallo, and C.M. Huang. "Antimicrobial Property of Lauric Acid against Propionibacterium Acnes: Its Therapeutic Potential for Inflammatory Acne Vulgaris." *Journal of Investigative Dermatology* 129, no. 10 (October 2009): 2480–88. doi:10.1038/jid.2009.93.

Nevin, K.G., and T. Rajamohan. "Effect of Topical Application of Virgin Coconut Oil on Skin Components and Antioxidant Status During Dermal Wound Healing in Young Rats." *Skin Pharmacology and Physiology* 23, no. 6 (2010): 290–97. doi:10.1159/000313516.

Nevin, K.G., and T. Rajamohan. "Beneficial Effects of Virgin Coconut Oil on Lipid Parameters and In Vitro LDL Oxidation." *Clinical Biochemistry* 37, no. 9 (September 2004): 830–35.

Nevin, K.G., and T. Rajamohan. "Influence of Virgin Coconut Oil on Blood Coagulation Factors, Lipid Levels and LDL Oxidation in Cholesterol-Fed Sprague–Dawley Rats." *European e-Journal of Clinical Nutrition and Metabolism* 3, no. 1 (February 2008): e1–e8.

Polo, Marco. *The Travels*. New York, NY: Signet, 2004.

Prior, I.A., F. Davidson, C.E. Salmond, and Z. Czochanska. "Cholesterol, Coconuts, and Diet on Polynesian Atolls: A Natural Experiment: The Pukapuka and Tokelau Island Studies." *American Journal of Clinical Nutrition* 34, no. 8 (August 1981): 1552–61.

Reger, M.A., S. T. Henderson, C. Hale, B. Cholerton, L. D. Baker, G.S. Watson, K. Hyde, et al. "Effects of Beta-Hydroxybutyrate on Cognition in Memory-Impaired Adults." *Neurobiology of Aging* 25, no. 3 (March 2004): 311–14.

Rego Costa, A.C., E.L. Rosado, and M. Soares-Mota. "Influence of the Dietary Intake of Medium Chain Triglycerides on Body Composition, Energy Expenditure and Satiety: A Systematic Review." *Nutrición Hospitalaria* 27, no. 1 (January 2012): 103–38. doi:10.1590/S0212-16112012000100011.

Rele, A.S. and R.B. Mohile. "Effect of Mineral Oil, Sunflower Oil, and Coconut Oil on Prevention of Hair Damage." *Journal of Cosmetic Science* 54, no. 2 (March 2003): 175–92.

Siri-Tarino, Patty W., Qi Sun, Frank B. Hu, and Ronald. M. Krauss. "Meta-analysis of Prospective Cohort Studies Evaluating the Association of Saturated Fat with Cardiovascular Disease." American Journal of Clinical Nutrition 91, no. 3 (March 2010): 535–546. doi: 10.3945/ajcn.2009.27725.

St-Onge, M.P. "Dietary Fats, Teas, Dairy, and Nuts: Potential Functional Foods for Weight Control?" *American Journal of Clinical Nutrition* 81, no. 1 (January 2005): 7–15.

St-Onge, M.P. and P.J. Jones. "Physiological Effects of Medium-Chain Triglycerides: Potential Agents in the Prevention of Obesity." *Journal of Nutrition* 132, no. 3 (March 2002): 329–32. doi:10.1024/0300-9831.78.6.275.

St-Onge, M.P., A. Bosarge, L.L.T. Goree, and B. Darnell. "Medium Chain Triglyceride Oil Consumption as Part of a Weight Loss Diet Does Not Lead to an Adverse Metabolic Profile When Compared to Olive Oil." *Journal of the American College of Nutrition* 27, no. 5 (2008): 547–552.

Vaidya, U.V., V.M. Hegde, S.A. Bhave, and A.N. Pandit. "Vegetable Oil Fortified Feeds in the Nutrition of Very Low Birthweight Babies." *Indian Pediatrics* 29, no 12 (December 1992): 1519–27.

Verallo-Rowell, V.M., K.M. Dillague, and B.S. Syah-Tjundawan. "Novel Antibacterial and Emollient Effects of Coconut and Virgin Olive Oils in Adult Atopic Dermatitis." *Dermatitis*. 19, no. 6 (November 2008): 308–15.

Villars, Teri. "Coconuts Saved Many Lives During Gas Attacks in World War I." *Hub Pages*, January 24, 2014. Accessed February 17, 2015. tvyps.hubpages.com/hub/gas-in-ww1.

Wang X., L. Pan, P. Zhang, X. Liu, G. Wu, Y. Wang, Y. Liu, et al. "Enteral Nutrition Improves Clinical Outcome and Shortens Hospital Stay After Cancer Surgery." *Journal of Investigative Surgery* 23, no. 6 (December 2010): 309–13. doi:10.3109/08941939.2010.519428.

Yeap, S. K., B.K. Beh, N.M. Ali, H.M. Yusof, W.Y. Ho, S.P. Koh, B Noorjahan, et al. "Antistress and Antioxidant Effects of Virgin Coconut Oil in Vivo." *Journal of Experimental and Therapeutic Medicine* 9, no. 1: (2015) 39–42. doi:10.3892/etm.2014.2045.

APPENDIX A
CONVERSION TABLES

VOLUME EQUIVALENTS (LIQUID)

US STANDARD	US STANDARD (OUNCES)	METRIC (APPROXIMATE)
2 tablespoons	1 fl. oz.	30 mL
¼ cup	2 fl. oz.	60 mL
½ cup	4 fl. oz.	120 mL
1 cup	8 fl. oz.	240 mL
1½ cups	12 fl. oz.	355 mL
2 cups or 1 pint	16 fl. oz.	475 mL
4 cups or 1 quart	32 fl. oz.	1 L
1 gallon	128 fl. oz.	4 L

OVEN TEMPERATURES

FAHRENHEIT (F)	CELSIUS (C) (APPROXIMATE)
250°	120°
300°	150°
325°	165°
350°	180°
375°	190°
400°	200°
425°	220°
450°	230°

VOLUME EQUIVALENTS (DRY)

US STANDARD	METRIC (APPROXIMATE)
⅛ teaspoon	0.5 mL
¼ teaspoon	1 mL
½ teaspoon	2 mL
¾ teaspoon	4 mL
1 teaspoon	5 mL
1 tablespoon	15 mL
¼ cup	59 mL
⅓ cup	79 mL
½ cup	118 mL
⅔ cup	156 mL
¾ cup	177 mL
1 cup	235 mL
2 cups or 1 pint	475 mL
3 cups	700 mL
4 cups or 1 quart	1 L

WEIGHT EQUIVALENTS

US STANDARD	METRIC (APPROXIMATE)
½ ounce	15 g
1 ounce	30 g
2 ounces	60 g
4 ounces	115 g
8 ounces	225 g
12 ounces	340 g
16 ounces or 1 pound	455 g

APPENDIX B
THE DIRTY DOZEN
& THE CLEAN FIFTEEN

A nonprofit environmental watchdog organization called Environmental Working Group (EWG) looks at data supplied by the US Department of Agriculture (USDA) and the Food and Drug Administration (FDA) about pesticide residues. Each year it compiles a list of the best and worst pesticide loads found in commercial crops. You can use these lists to decide which fruits and vegetables to buy organic to minimize your exposure to pesticides and which produce is considered safe enough to buy conventionally. This does not mean they are pesticide-free, though, so wash these fruits and vegetables thoroughly.

These lists change every year, so make sure you look up the most recent one before you fill your shopping cart. You'll find the most recent lists as well as a guide to pesticides in produce at EWG.org/FoodNews.

2015 Dirty Dozen

Apples	Peaches	*In addition to the Dirty Dozen, the EWG added two types of produce contaminated with highly toxic organo-phosphate insecticides:*
Celery	Potatoes	
Cherry tomatoes	Snap peas (imported)	
Cucumbers	Spinach	
Grapes	Strawberries	Kale/Collard greens
Nectarines (imported)	Sweet bell peppers	Hot peppers

2015 Clean Fifteen

Asparagus	Eggplants	Papayas
Avocados	Grapefruits	Pineapples
Cabbage	Kiwis	Sweet corn
Cantaloupes (domestic)	Mangoes	Sweet peas (frozen)
Cauliflower	Onions	Sweet potatoes

RECIPE INDEX

INDEX

TEN PALEO RECIPES

From the Best-Selling Book *Paleo for Beginners*

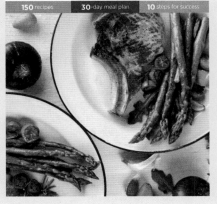

Also by Sonoma Press

If you enjoy the delicious, nourishing recipes in *The Coconut Oil Cure*, then you'll love the 150 easy recipes in *Paleo for Beginners*. The Paleo diet cuts out unhealthful modern foods like grains, sugars, and processed products, and replaces them with only the freshest, healthiest, and most nutrient-packed foods. In addition to recipes that take advantage of the health benefits of coconut oil, apple cider vinegar, and other beneficial ingredients, *Paleo for Beginners* offers a 30-day meal plan to help you get lean and feel more energetic.

Available from Sonoma Press wherever books are sold.

Italian Vegetable Frittata

MAKES 4 SERVINGS

Artichoke hearts play a pivotal role in this festive frittata. These tasty flower buds are a great source of antioxidants and fiber. Artichoke hearts can decrease the risk of certain types of cancer and cardiovascular disease. Try to find hearts packed in water if you don't want to steam or blanch fresh artichokes.

2 cups egg whites (about 20 egg whites)

½ cup freshly shredded vegan cheese

2 tablespoons chopped fresh basil

Cracked black pepper to taste

1 teaspoon olive oil

1 teaspoon minced garlic

2 scallions, finely chopped

½ cup canned quartered artichoke hearts, drained

1 cup halved cherry or grape tomatoes

1 ounce diced, lean nitrate-free ham

1. Preheat oven to broil.

2. In a medium bowl, whisk together the egg whites, cheese, basil, and pepper; set aside.

3. Place a large ovenproof skillet over medium-high heat; add the olive oil. Add the garlic and scallions and sauté for 1 minute.

4. Add the artichoke hearts, tomatoes, and ham and saute for 3 to 4 minutes.

5. Remove the skillet from heat and pour in the egg mixture.

6. Return the skillet to the heat, cover, and cook without stirring for 10 to 12 minutes, or until the egg mixture is set in center.

7. Remove from the heat and place under skillet under the broiler for 1 minute or until the top is lightly browned.

8. Transfer to a serving plate and cut into quarters. Serve hot or at room temperature.

Chocolate-Raspberry Donuts

MAKES 6 DONUTS

Did you ever think you would be eating donuts while following a Paleo diet plan? With a donut pan you can create these dense treats easily—and they are Paleo! Donut pans can be found in most kitchen or baking supplies stores and online. You can create a simple chocolate glaze by melting a little dark chocolate with coconut oil and drizzling it over the cooled donuts.

Coconut oil, for greasing the pan

2 cups fine almond meal

¼ cup unsweetened cocoa powder

2 teaspoons coconut flour

1 teaspoon baking soda

Pinch of sea salt

4 large eggs

¼ cup honey

¼ cup coconut oil

1 teaspoon pure vanilla extract

1 cup fresh raspberries

⅓ cup dark chocolate chips

1. Preheat the oven to 350°F. Lightly grease a donut pan with coconut oil.

2. In a large bowl, stir together the almond meal, cocoa, coconut flour, baking soda, and salt until well combined.

3. In a medium bowl, whisk together the eggs, honey, coconut oil, and vanilla.

4. Add the wet ingredients to the dry ingredients and stir to mix well.

5. Carefully fold in the raspberries and chocolate chips.

6. Spoon the batter into the donut pan and tap lightly on the counter to remove air bubbles.

7. Bake for 20 to 25 minutes, until firm.

8. Let cool and serve.

Citrus Poached Salmon

MAKES 4 SERVINGS

You can make this fish recipe the day or evening before to enjoy for a quick lunch the next day. Salmon is valued nutritionally because it is a great source of omega-3 fatty acids, which help reduce the risk of many cardiovascular problems, improve brain health, and decrease inflammation in the joints. Purchase certified wild salmon whenever possible, and keep in mind that there are contamination issues associated with some farmed fish.

8 cups water

⅓ cup fresh lemon juice

1 small yellow onion, sliced

1 garlic clove, crushed

1 large carrot, peeled and thinly sliced

1 cup celery leaves, coarsely chopped

1 tablespoon chopped fresh thyme

1 teaspoon cracked black pepper

1 teaspoon chopped fresh dill

2 bay leaves

½ teaspoon sea salt

4 (8-ounce) salmon fillets

1. Place all the ingredients except the salmon fillets in a large pot and bring to a boil.

2. Immediately reduce the heat to low and gently simmer the liquid for about 1 hour.

3. Remove from the heat and cool the poaching liquid for about 10 minutes.

4. Strain the liquid through a fine sieve or a piece of cheesecloth into a large, wide skillet; discard the solids.

5. Place the skillet over low heat and bring the poaching liquid to a gentle simmer.

6. Carefully add the salmon fillets in one layer.

7. Cover the skillet and simmer the salmon for about 10 minutes, or until it looks opaque and is just cooked through.

8. Remove the salmon fillets carefully from the liquid and let them cool completely.

9. Serve the poached salmon with fresh sliced cucumbers or your favorite salad.

Shrimp and Peach Tostadas

MAKES 4 SERVINGS

This is the perfect dish for a relaxed lunch on a sunny patio with friends, accompanied by a refreshing pitcher of tart lemonade. The tortillas are crisp, the shrimp savory, and the peach salsa is sweet and hot. You can also substitute mango, plums, or papaya for the peaches if you want a different taste sensation.

1 tablespoon olive oil

1 teaspoon minced garlic

½ pound medium shrimp, shelled
    and deveined

4 Paleo tortillas

Juice of 2 limes

1 ripe peach, pitted and diced

1 small red bell pepper, julienned

½ cup chopped chives

1 jalapeño pepper, seeded and minced

½ teaspoon salt

2 cups shredded romaine lettuce

½ cup plain vegan yogurt

1. Preheat oven to 375°F.

2. Place the olive oil in a large skillet over medium-high heat and sauté the garlic for 1 minute.

3. Add the shrimp to the skillet and sauté until it is pink and opaque, about 2 minutes.

4. Remove the shrimp and place it into a bowl to cool with some ice.

5. Place the tortillas on a baking sheet and bake in the oven for about 10 minutes, turning halfway through, until crisp.

6. Drain the shrimp and discard any ice that is left in the bowl. Add the lime juice, chopped peach, red pepper, chives, jalapeño pepper, and salt to the shrimp and toss to combine.

7. Top the crisp tortillas with the shredded romaine lettuce and then the shrimp mixture.

8. Serve with a small dollop of vegan yogurt.

Almond Butter Cups

MAKES 16 CUPS

Anyone who likes peanut butter cups will love these tasty treats. Homemade almond butter is the best choice, but an organic product is fine as long as it contains no sugar. To get the perfect double dark and light layers, make sure the bottom layer is completely chilled before adding the dark chocolate on top. If the topping gets too firm, remelt it.

2 cups dark chocolate, chopped

1 cup almond butter

Pinch of sea salt

½ cup chopped almonds

1. In a medium bowl placed over a pot of gently simmering water, melt the chocolate, stirring constantly.

2. Remove half of the melted chocolate to a container and stir in the almond butter and the salt until smooth.

3. Spoon the almond butter mixture into paper candy cups, filling them about half full. Place them in the fridge until hardened, at least 1 hour.

4. Remelt the plain dark chocolate, if necessary, and spoon it evenly over the chilled almond cups.

5. Place them back in the fridge until completely chilled, about 1 hour.

6. Store the almond cups in the freezer in a sealed container.

Herbed Beef Jerky

MAKES 6 SERVINGS

Any kind of jerky is very simple to make at home with either an oven or a dehydrator. The trick to getting great long-lasting jerky that will not spoil is to start with very lean meat completely trimmed of fat. This recipe can also be made using other meats such as buffalo, elk, or venison.

2 teaspoons onion salt

¾ teaspoon cracked black pepper

¾ teaspoon dried oregano

½ teaspoon sea salt

½ teaspoon garlic powder

½ teaspoon dried thyme

½ teaspoon dried basil

2 pounds lean steak, fat trimmed and cut into ¼-inch strips

1. Preheat the oven to the lowest possible temperature. Line two backing sheets with aluminum foil.

2. In a small bowl, mix together all the herbs, spices, salt, and pepper until well blended.

3. Arrange the beef strips on a cutting board and rub half the spice mixture into the meat. Pound the meat with a mallet to work the spice mixture in deeply.

4. Turn all the strips over and repeat the process with the rest of the spice mixture.

5. Transfer the strips to the prepared baking sheets, placing them in a single layer, and put them in the oven with the door propped open.

6. Leave the beef strips in the oven for about 8 hours to dry, and then flip them over and dry them on the other side for 8 hours.

7. Store the jerky in an airtight container at room temperature.

Chicken Shepherd's Pie

MAKES 6 SERVINGS

Traditional shepherd's pie usually features ground beef and mashed potatoes, so this tasty sweet potato–topped chicken variation makes a nice variation. The trick to a truly successful shepherd's pie is to completely cook the meat portion of the dish. Top this savory mixture with the mashed sweet potatoes and reheat in the oven until the top is lightly browned and bubbling.

3 large sweet potatoes, peeled and cut into chunks
½ teaspoon olive oil
1 small onion, chopped
2 cups button mushrooms, cut in quarters
2 teaspoons minced garlic
2 cups low-sodium chicken stock
3 tablespoons water

2 tablespoons arrowroot starch
3 poached chicken breasts cut into medium chunks
2 carrots, peeled and cut into thin disks and blanched until tender
2 cups fresh peas
2 teaspoon minced fresh thyme
Sea salt and cracked black pepper to taste

1. Preheat oven to 350°F.

2. Boil the sweet potatoes until very soft; drain and mash, then set aside.

3. Heat the oil in a large skillet, and sauté the onion, mushrooms, and garlic until softened, about 5 minutes.

4. Add the stock to the skillet and heat to a simmer over medium heat.

5. In a small bowl, whisk the water and arrowroot together until there are no lumps.

6. Pour the arrowroot mixture into simmering stock mixture. Stir until the sauce is thick.

7. Add the chicken, carrots, peas, and thyme to the skillet and stir to combine. Season with salt and pepper.

8. Spoon the chicken mixture into a large baking dish and spread the mashed sweet potatoes over the top, completely covering the chicken mixture.

9. Bake until the filling bubbles along the edges, about 35 minutes.

Pork Chops with Spiced Apples and Thyme

MAKES 4 SERVINGS

Have you ever wondered whether the saying, "an apple a day keeps the doctor away," is true? Well, there is truth in this old folk remedy. Apples are one of the healthiest foods available, especially if organic. They are a great source of soluble fiber called pectin, which makes apples very effective at controlling blood sugar, reducing the risk of many cancers, and lowering cholesterol. This recipe is best with tart varieties of apples to accent the thyme and cinnamon.

1 teaspoon olive oil

4 boneless pork chops, fat trimmed

1 small sweet onion, thinly sliced

2 large tart apples with their skin, cored and sliced thinly

½ cup apple juice

1 tablespoon whole grain Dijon mustard

1 teaspoon chopped fresh thyme

½ teaspoon ground cinnamon

Sea salt and cracked black pepper to taste

1. Preheat oven to 350°F.

2. Heat the olive oil in a large ovenproof skillet over medium heat. Add the pork chops and brown on both sides. Remove the pork chops from the skillet and set aside on a plate.

3. Add the onion to the skillet and sauté until softened, about 5 minutes.

4. Add the apple slices to the onions and sauté until the apples are softened, about 5 minutes.

5. Stir in the apple juice, mustard, thyme, and cinnamon.

6. Move the onion mixture to the side of the pan and return the pork chops to the pan along with any juices on the plate.

7. Spoon the onion mixture over the pork chops, cover, and place the skillet in the preheated oven. Cook until the pork chops are tender, about 35 minutes.

9. Season with salt and pepper, and serve hot.

Toffee Apples

These sticky, juicy treats will bring out the kid in anyone. Timing is crucial when making and chilling the caramel, because if it is too thick you will not be able to roll the apples in it. Make sure your apples are completely dry before applying the caramel or it will simply slip right off the fruit. If you cannot get the caramel to coat the apples evenly and neatly, don't despair; it also works as a delectable dip with crisp apple wedges.

2 cups raw cashews

¾ cup maple syrup

½ cup plus 2 tablespoons water

3 tablespoons coconut oil

1 tablespoon pure vanilla extract

Pinch of sea salt

8 firm tart apples, washed and stems removed

8 wooden candy apple sticks

1½ cups finely chopped nuts, optional

1. Place the cashews, maple syrup, water, coconut oil, and vanilla in a blender and process until very smooth. This is the caramel mixture.

2. Transfer the caramel to a deep medium bowl and place it in the fridge, covered, until the caramel is thick, 15 to 20 minutes.

3. Place the chopped nuts in another bowl.

4. For each apple, insert a wood stick three-quarters of the way through the bottom.

5. Dry the washed apples thoroughly with a paper towel.

6. Carefully dip the apples in the caramel so that they are completely covered, and then roll them in the nuts, if desired.

7. Place the finished apples on a plate and chill them standing up in the fridge until firm. Serve cold.

Molten Chocolate Lava Cake

MAKES 6 SERVINGS

What could be better than this tender chocolate cake oozing with rich chocolate sauce? They are very easy to make. You can serve them either in the ramekins or pop them out onto serving plates for a more elegant presentation. Garnish with fresh berries and mint. If using ramekins, lightly grease them with oil and dust with cocoa powder so the cakes don't stick.

Coconut oil for greasing the ramekins

5 ounces dark chocolate

5 tablespoons coconut oil

2 extra-large eggs

1 teaspoon pure vanilla extract

2 tablespoons maple syrup

Pinch of sea salt

2 teaspoons cocoa powder

1 teaspoon coconut flour

1. Preheat oven to 375°F. Lightly grease six 6-ounce ramekins with coconut oil.

2. Melt the chocolate and coconut oil carefully in the microwave until smooth, taking care not to burn it. Transfer to a medium bowl and cool for 15 minutes.

3. Whisk together the eggs, vanilla, maple syrup, and salt until light and frothy.

4. Add the egg mixture to the chocolate along with the cocoa and coconut flour. Fold to incorporate all the ingredients well.

5. Spoon the batter into the prepared ramekins so they are about half full.

6. Transfer the ramekins to a baking sheet and bake for 12 to15 minutes, until the edges are set, but the center is still soft.

7. Serve warm.

CONVERSION TABLES

OVEN TEMPERATURES	
CELSIUS (C)	FAHRENHEIT (F)
120	250
150	300
180	355
200	400
220	450

VOLUME EQUIVALENTS	
METRIC	IMPERIAL (APPROXIMATE)
20 ML	½ FL OZ
60 ML	2 FL OZ
80 ML	3 FL OZ
125 ML	4 ½ FL OZ
160 ML	5 ½ FL OZ
180 ML	6 FL OZ
250 ML	9 FL OZ
375 ML	13 FL OZ
500 ML	18 FL OZ
750 ML	1 ½ PINTS
1 LITRE	1 ¾ PINTS

WEIGHT EQUIVALENTS	
METRIC	IMPERIAL (APPROXIMATE)
10 G	⅓ OZ
50 G	2 OZ
80 G	3 OZ
100 G	3 ½ OZ
150 G	5 OZ
175 G	6 OZ
250 G	9 OZ
375 G	13 OZ
500 G	1 LB
750 G	1 ⅔ LB
1 KG	2 LB

CUP AND SPOON CONVERSIONS	
5 ML	1 TEASPOON
20 ML	1 TABLESPOON
60 ML	¼ CUP
80 ML	⅓ CUP
125 ML	½ CUP
160 ML	⅔ CUP
180 ML	¾ CUP
250 ML	1 CUP